"Should've Died When You Were Born!"

Anna Maria Scott

"Should've Died When You Were Born!"
Copyright © 2024 by Anna Maria Scott

All rights reserved. No part of this publication may be reproduced, distributed, or transmitted in any form or by any means, including photocopying, recording, or other electronic or mechanical methods, without the prior written permission of the author, except in the case of brief quotations embodied in critical reviews and certain other non-commercial uses permitted by copyright law.

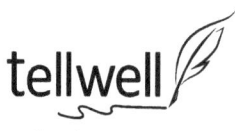

Tellwell Talent
www.tellwell.ca

ISBN
978-0-2288-9356-1 (Hardcover)
978-0-2288-9355-4 (Paperback)
978-0-2288-9357-8 (eBook)

Prologue

WITH NO HOPE ON THE HORIZON

I grappled with thoughts of suicide

as I sped along the highway blinded

by tears…

I'll just slam into the next pole!!

Too late!…the next one then!!

Chapter 1

I can only imagine what my mother was thinking and feeling after she gave birth to me and the doctor announced, "There's another one in there!"

Twins are usually born within minutes of each other, but my identical twin didn't arrive until two hours and fifteen minutes later. My mother had already given birth to thirteen children, one of which died soon after being born, and had a miscarriage with twins before we arrived, so it's fair to say that she was not overly excited about bringing—not one, but two!—more babies into the world that day.

I was given the name Anna and my twin sister was named Anita.

It was December 21, 1942, in the coal mining town of New Waterford, Cape Breton, Nova Scotia. Population around 10,000. My father owned a meat and grocery business on Plummer Avenue (the main street in town) that was doing exceedingly well. Our house was situated near the top of a hill just off the main street, a couple of minutes' walk from home.

My father, whom we called Papa, spent most of his time at the store. He was an easy-going type of a person. Six feet tall, of average build, with a bald spot showing on the top of his head when he wasn't wearing his hat that matched his grey suit. I remember how he would occasionally take Anita and I on his knee when we were just toddlers and talk to us in a very soothing tone, as if trying to make us feel wanted. Taking his gold watch with a chain attached from his vest pocket, he would make conversation around that, for example. And at night time whenever I couldn't sleep, I would go to his side of the bed to wake him up. He would always take my hand, and leading me back to my room would whisper, "The angels are waiting at the top of the bed." Ever so gently, he would cover Anita and I as he lovingly tucked us in, saying, "Back to back."

My mother, we called her Mama, on the other hand, was the complete opposite as far as expressing any kind of emotion. Never did we feel the warmth of a mother's hug or hear the words "I love you." We constantly felt rejected and like we were nothing but a bother to her.

The Catholic Church was the centre of her life, and the fear of going to hell dominated her thinking. Every Sunday she would faithfully attend Mass, proudly dressed with her stylish hat and gloves. Anita and I walked on either side, also wearing hats, gloves, and ribbons in our neatly braided hair.

Although soft spoken, Mama was always firm on one thing: we were to be "obedient." She was swift with the hand, and a slap in the face would put us in our place in an instant. Kids should be seen but not heard was the understanding, and any questions were ignored. Any attempt to express our feelings or concerns were also disregarded. Growing up with this mentality meant we didn't understand what a healthy, normal interaction was. The little things most children take for granted, like celebrating their birthday with cake, candles and friends singing "Happy Birthday," was not something I experienced.

I can only *imagine* what my mother was thinking and feeling as she gave birth to us because she did not want children but had them only out of a sense of duty. Each pregnancy must have been very difficult to accept. Within a span of twenty years she gave birth to fifteen children. Of the fourteen of us who survived, there were seven boys and seven girls.

I can remember our parish priest Father Campbell at the pulpit asking the congregation, "How many children should you have? As many as God will give you." Birth control of any kind was not allowed in the Catholic Church, so in retrospect I can empathize not only with my mother's situation but with all those women who had to live under that kind of conditioning.

"Should've Died When You Were Born!"

I have this rather vague memory of Mama saying that she had worn a corset during her last pregnancy while carrying Anita and I so that no one could tell she was pregnant. She had given birth to all the previous babies in the hospital, but she decided to have a home delivery for the last one. Apparently, someone had remarked that she was like a baby factory. Even though large families were common at the time, she was self-conscious and a very proud person, so the comment must have stung. She was ashamed to be in that condition once again, so she wanted to give birth at home.

That's when she received the hugely disappointing news that two babies were on the way! The doctor suggested she go into the hospital to have a tubal ligation after we were born, which she agreed to. She was forty-five years old, and I'm sure she must have been terribly guilt ridden because of her strict religious background. At the same time, it must have been a huge relief to know there would no more pregnancies.

Our older siblings who had left home for either Montreal or Toronto would come home occasionally for very short visits, so we never did get to know them. None of my brothers had ever worked in the coal mines, and the ones that stayed in New Waterford worked for Papa. Frankie, one of my brothers, had his little bungalow on the next street over from our house and worked in the store as the butcher. Another brother named Willie delivered groceries for Papa.

My earliest memories are of us being in two large ivory-coloured metal cribs just outside Mama's room in the hallway upstairs. My older brother Louis mentioned that Anita and I were never taken outside of the house until we were two years old. I understand that Mama had hurt her ankle and was bedridden for a short time, and when the doctor came to attend to her ankle and saw us there in the cribs, he pointed out to her that we should be taken outside to get some sun and fresh air. So that was when they decided to rent a cabin in Catalone, and we spent that whole summer in the fresh country air.

I clearly remember my very first trip in the car. When I became startled by the sudden loud sound of the engine starting up, I began to cry, and when it started to move, I was terrified as the earth appeared to be moving outside the window. But what also comes to mind is the freedom we felt just being outside for the first time and surrounded by all that greenery with the peaceful sound of the water lapping at the waters' edge. These are beautiful memories I will always cherish.

Preparing for bedtime in the soft glow of the lantern, there was a comforting feeling of peace and serenity in the room. I'd fall asleep inhaling that pure, fresh air that wafted in through the window next to me. In the morning, I woke up to the sound of birds chirping and the warm sun streaming into the room. I couldn't wait to get outside to feel the cool, soft grass beneath my feet. Whenever we'd hear a short *Toot! Toot!* coming from the steam train that slowly made its way along the tracks, we'd run down the slight embankment in front of the veranda to pick up the *Cape Breton Post* that was tossed out along the way. I fell in love with nature that first summer at the lake in Catalone, and to this day whenever I am out in the country, I love that special healing effect from mother earth. It always takes my mind to a deeper level of appreciation for all of creation.

Whenever Anita and I walked the short distance from our house to our store on Plummer Avenue, Papa would often ask us to go a few doors over to another store, called Harrisons', where he bought his pencils and White Owl cigars. We would always ask him for some extra money so we could buy our favourite caramel candies while we were there. When he opened the cash register, the drawer would pop open with a loud *cling!* and he'd hand one of us a nickel and the other a dime. He'd always wait for our reaction, which was always the same.

"Oh no, I want the bigger one like she has," the one with the dime would say.

He'd laugh and give us both the same size coin, then off we'd go happily thinking that the bigger coins (the nickels) were worth more than the dimes.

One day, for whatever reason Anita and I decided to take another route home from the store instead of the usual one. I see us standing on the sidewalk in front of a big grey stone church on a hill of a street we were not familiar with. We were talking to a friendly little girl around our age when she asked if we'd like to see her dolls. She led us around to the back of the church and into the basement and happily showed us her dolls that were in her "playroom" as she called it. When we got home, Mama asked where we were because we had been gone awhile. When we told her about our little adventure, which was only two blocks away from home, she scolded us and said we were not to play with that little girl. I was so surprised! She said the girl was the daughter of the minister of that church and because we were Catholic, we shouldn't go there. Maybe she was afraid we would be converted? I don't know. But in her mind, she must have thought she was protecting us somehow.

I must say that I do not regret having to go to church on Sundays. Actually I liked to hear the stories about Christ and how he taught people about love and forgiveness. I never had any fear of God growing up, and I appreciate Christ's teachings even more now as an adult, especially since I chose the spiritual path of yoga meditation in my early thirties. When I left the church, it was not Christ I was turning away from but rather from the Church's hierarchy. I was never comfortable with it, and I finally rejected it altogether.

The only area in our town that Anita and I were familiar with as we grew up was between our house, our store on Plummer Ave and the church and school we attended. All were within walking distance of each other. There were other parishes in our town as well, but they seemed rather foreign to us. Our world was very small indeed.

Our house on Mahon Street, which was just off of Plummer Avenue, had a large field extending all the way over to the next street, called Saint Anne. There was a long one-storey barn for the team of horses, named Molly and Peggy, as well as a grey pony named Peanuts that belonged to our brother Tony. At one end of the barn were the horses' stalls, and in the middle was a large room with high-stacked bundles of hay. At the other end was a cement floor with enough space to hold a fancy red wagon with large, thin wheels, along with a jeep and station wagon. A gas pump was at the entrance, which bordered on Saint-Anne Street.

Anita and I used to walk through the back yard to get to our store on Plummer Ave. We found people to be very friendly, often commenting on how cute we looked as we walked hand in hand. We were not the only set of twins in town; there were the Dr. Miller twins as well. They lived in a huge house with black shingles and white trim on the main street, just a few doors over from our store. We were allowed to go there and spend time with the twins, Charles and Anne, who were a bit younger than us. We enjoyed playing in their backyard, which felt more like a park because they had swings with thick chains and a big wooden see-saw that moved around in a circle.

Anita and I were on their see-saw one day when she happened to be on the end that was up high and I must have inadvertently let go or whatever, so she suddenly came crashing down with one big thud. I was alarmed because she was slumped over the wooden handle, not moving.

"ANITA! ARE YOU OKAY?"

I tried to help her up, but she was moaning as if in pain.

"Here, hang onto me," I said as I put one arm around her waist while trying to hold her up with the other.

It was clear she had injured herself, so I wanted to get her home as quickly as possible. She started sobbing from the pain when I had to practically drag her along.

When we reached the house, I called out for Mama to come and help.

"Oh just put her on the couch there in the dining room," she said, turning away.

She did not want to know what had happened. I managed to get Anita onto the couch at least, where she eventually fell asleep. She said that when she woke up, she wasn't able to stand up because of the pain. She had to spend the entire night there, afraid and shivering in the dark, unable to move. We knew it was useless to mention it the next day to Mama because she had already showed she didn't want to hear about it. I don't remember how long it took Anita to recover, but she had a sort of limp for quite a while after that fall.

Our older sisters Justine and Adeline both happened to be engaged to be married when Anita and I were around five years old. Once in a while, when Justine was sitting with George in his car parked in the yard, we'd ask if we could get in the back. They didn't seem to mind. One day, Adeline's boyfriend Wilfred also had his truck parked near the back step. He was inside the house with Adeline, so Anita and I decided to climb into the back, which was open with a sheet of plywood on either side. We thought we'd hide there so that when Wilfred came out, we'd get to go back to his place with him. We liked him a lot, and we'd get away from Mama for a while. Anyway, there we were, hiding, when Wilfred came out and started the truck and left. He drove home to Lingan, which is on the edge of New Waterford without noticing us. When we were discovered, nobody was amused, and, to our disappointment, Wilfred had to bring us right back home.

When our brother Tony, who is two years older than Anita and I, started going to school, I wanted to go too. I simply wanted to get out of the house since the feeling of not being wanted by Mama never lifted from day one. Everyone started school at age six in those days, so our older sister Justine was told to take us. She did and then returned to take us home again on the first day. However, on the second day, we found ourselves coming home after school all alone. Anita and I were taking our time as we strolled along a wide brook when we suddenly realized we had lost our way! Some people must have noticed us wandering because they came over and asked us some questions. We knew they were trying to be helpful when they guided us back to the main street and onto the sidewalk. That's where we recognized the large grey building at the corner of the street with the name "Eaton" on it, so were able to find our way home from there. I was always easily confused when not in our familiar surroundings, so home was a safe place to be even though we never felt accepted or wanted by Mama.

A memory just popped up in my mind of being with Justine, our older sister, when I was probably around six years old. I don't know where we were, the image is not very clear, but it's what happened emotionally that stands out in my mind. As we were about to get into a vehicle that looked like a minibus that had pulled up in front of us, I suddenly became overwhelmed with this horrible feeling that if I got inside I wouldn't be able to breathe—I would be trapped! I actually thought I was going to die! So as Justine took my hand with the intention of helping me to get in, I quickly let go and pulled away from her. She became impatient when I started to cry while resisting with all my might.

"NO!" I screamed.

She and the driver hadn't a clue what was going through my mind, of course. She finally let go of me when she saw there was no way I was going to get inside. I'm sure she was terribly embarrassed and annoyed with having to deal with me. She had no idea I was reacting out of a fear that came from God knows where that day.

I also remember another incident, but the circumstances are clear with this one. It was in the beginning of our first year of school, maybe just a few days after school started. Anita and I were outside in the schoolyard at recess time watching the other children singing and playing a game called "London Bridge is Falling Down." One of the teachers tried to get us to join in, but I was too shy and I squeezed Anita's hand as a signal for us to back off. So we simply stood by as they continued on with their game. We never spoke much, even to each other, as we grew up; we just seemed to know somehow what the other one was thinking. Most likely because we had shared the womb together.

Anyway, I remember always observing others instead of taking part in whatever was going on. One day when our teacher, who was a nun, was leading us in the morning prayer, I saw that the other students were not aware that she began to act in a very strange manner. She started pacing back and forth with a rather nervous energy, then suddenly burst into tears. We were all surprised, and confusion set in. A couple of the children began to cry, and as I sat in stunned silence watching, another nun appeared at the door within seconds, demanding that the hysterical nun "Calm down!" Instead, the frantic nun pushed the intruding nun back while trying to close the door on her. Next thing I knew we were quickly being ushered into a dimly lit hallway where someone helped us find our coats and we were quickly led outside of the building. It was, and still is, a puzzle to me what caused the nun to break down as she did that day. I wonder whatever happened to her?

The nuns, who were called the Sisters of Charity, lived in a large convent right next to the school. Most of them were our teachers, but when I entered Grade 2, I happened to have a woman teacher instead of a nun. I remember her standing up in front of us saying that we were not to talk to anyone while in class. I was distracted by this little girl I admired who was sitting directly in front of me. I just loved her thick, golden braids and the beautiful crocheted light blue and pink sweater she was wearing. I wanted to tell her what I was thinking and began whispering to her. I was startled to hear my name called out and the teacher directing me to come up in front of the class. I didn't have a clue as to what she wanted, but I did as I was told. I was puzzled when I saw her reaching for a long, thick, greyish strap on her desk. She ordered me to hold out my hand. I was shocked as she lifted her hand up high and struck me once with one quick hard *whack!* She said I was not to talk to others during class! It stung, but I was mostly stunned! I felt my face turn red with shame and could feel everyone's eyes on me as I walked back to my desk. I just wanted to run out the door and never go back!

When Louis, my brother who is seventeen years older than Anita and I, came home on a rare visit from Montreal, he brought some beautiful gold satin drapes for our living room, or "parlour" as they called it in those days. He had expensive taste for clothes, as did Mama, and, like her, he enjoyed playing the piano, which became his passion later on in life. He also brought two sets of dolls. One set, called the soldier dolls, were about twelve inches high and wearing green berets and shorts. I understood they were meant to sit on both sides of the fire place as ornaments. The other set were cute girl dolls about eighteen inches high with pretty dresses and bonnets that were meant for us to play with. For some reason, Mama decided both sets should be placed on each side of the fireplace. So we could only look at them through the glass squares of the French doors, which were locked except for when she had visitors or when she went in to play the piano.

During the Christmas season, though, the doors were opened and a large Christmas tree was placed between the dining room and parlour. We had gotten used to not touching the dolls, so we eventually forgot about them and our interest turned to our shiny black piano instead. Mama and Louis played, and Anita and I enjoyed singing the songs that scrolled down when you pumped the pedals. They were mainly Christmas songs like "Let it snow." The keys moved up and down as if someone was actually playing the piano.

Chapter 2

So there were nice memories, too, and now as I look back, I don't think Mama was intentionally being mean or heartless when she ignored our emotional needs. She didn't seem to comprehend we had feelings and that all children need to be nurtured and loved in order to grow into healthy, functioning human beings. A couple of times she mentioned that someone had made a comment regarding her motherly skills (or lack thereof, I should say) and seemed proud to quote what was said: "Jenny you should have been a nun!" I understood what the person meant because it was obvious when she'd demonstrate such a lack of sensitivity towards us. But we were so used to it we thought it was normal and that it was the same in other families as well.

However, I began to notice that other children our age had completely different relationships with their mothers than we had with ours, and at times I couldn't help but feel a little envious whenever I'd witness a loving bond between them. Anita and I happened to be walking home from school with a classmate one day when she invited us into her home. We were probably around seven or eight at the time. Not only was she greeted warmly by her mother who showed genuine interest in how her day went at school, but she praised her work as well. That moment of interaction between her and her mother left a lasting impression in my mind. I began to wonder what it was about Anita and I that caused Mama to disconnect from us the way she did. So whenever I'd see a mother actually talking to or showing the slightest interest in her child after that, I have to admit I was jealous and began to resent having to go home. More often than not, Mama would have something negative to say that let us know we were not wanted.

One day when Anita I came in from school and she just happened to be ironing the red ribbons for our hair, she said, "You know? If I didn't have you two, I could be out travelling like Mrs. MacDonald," (they owned the hardware and lumber store in town).

She'd also come up with remarks like, "Why can't you be like Marion?" our cousin who was studying to be a nurse. "Her mother is so proud of her!"

Every once in a while, she would remind us that we were simply a bother. She would blurt out things like that whenever she became impatient with us. One time when Anita and I wanted to go outside in the rain, she said "No! People will think I'm crazy to let you go out in this weather!" I guess I was the one brazen enough to come back and ask again, but then she suddenly grabbed the poker next to the stove and shaking it at us in anger said, "should've died when you were born!"

We both ran from the kitchen like scared little rabbits. I had a pair of long brown stockings in my hand as I dove behind a large armchair to hide. One of the socks got caught on the back and was left hanging there—giving me away, I thought. But when I felt it was safe enough to come out a couple of minutes later, both Mama and Anita had disappeared. I put my stocking on, wondering where they went. I found Anita upstairs getting ready to go outside. Apparently Mama had changed her mind because the next thing I remember is being outside with rubber boots on, walking through grassy puddles in our field, singing a song that was popular at the time.

Just walking in the rain
Thinking how we met
People come to windows
They always stare at me
Shake their heads in sorrow
Saying, "Who can that fool be?"

It's funny because when Mama said people would think she's crazy to allow us to go out in the rain, I believed they were now thinking I must be crazy because there I was outside just walking in the rain.

We rarely asked questions because we knew that any spark of curiosity would be extinguished, so we were in the dark about what was going on at home. I can vividly recall the day when Papa had to go away and how surprised I was—he was always there in our store. We found out later that he had an eye condition that needed immediate attention, so he had to fly to Montreal to have surgery. He had actually lost sight in one eye and was told it had to be removed. He was slowly losing sight in the other one as well. Since he had no warning signs, he was unaware he had a serious problem until it was too late.

While he was in surgery in Montreal, someone stole his expensive watch and ring. Although the operation itself went well, he was told nothing could be done to prevent the other eye from deteriorating, so he had to accept the fact that he would eventually be blind.

He wore a light pink plastic shield over the area of his missing eye and went back to working in the store as usual.

I don't know exactly when, but Papa started to have financial difficulties with his business. I became aware of this when I happened to be out on our back step one day as he was coming home from the store through the backyard, as usual. He was obviously very disturbed and trying to hide it when he passed by. He entered the house without saying anything, which was strange. I stayed in the porch with the door slightly open, listening out of sheer curiosity. Since I had never seen him in that state of mind before, I was concerned and surprised when he suddenly demanded, "Where's the station wagon?! Where's the station wagon?!" He said that customers were calling for their grocery orders that were supposed to have been delivered a long time ago. Since I'd never heard arguments—or even loud voices—in our home before, I was taken aback when I heard him shout like that in anger.

I opened the door a little more and peeked through.

I slowly moved into the kitchen where I could see him standing in the hallway at the bottom of the stairs. I must have felt his frustration because I remember feeling so sorry for him. I could see he was unable to control himself, and I felt helpless to do or say anything. This was so out of character for him! There was no response from whomever he was shouting to upstairs, so he turned back towards the kitchen. He didn't see me quickly slip back into the porch and out the back door, where I disappeared around the corner of the house. From there I saw him head back towards the store in a huff.

I could not stop myself as I ran towards the store after he was out of sight. When I got there, I opened the door, slowly trying to enter without being noticed. He was standing next to the desk in his office talking on the phone; he was still very upset. When my brother Frankie the butcher saw me, I turned and casually walked over to the fruit that was displayed in the front window of the store and picked up an orange, pretending that's what I had come in for.

When he went on with what he was doing, I crouched down and slowly crept along behind the meat counter towards Papa's office. I was anxious to know what was happening with him. But as Frankie came around the counter and opened the big heavy door to the refrigerated room, he spotted me in the corner of his eye.

"What are you doing here!" he said angrily.

In those few blinks when the door to the cold room was open, I caught a glimpse of the large, skinned animals hanging from shiny silver hooks. The image is still clear in my mind. I did not know then that it was the carcasses from which the butcher cuts the steaks and roasts we were served at mealtime.

"I want to talk to Papa!" I blurted.

"No, he's busy! Go home!"

I reluctantly gave in and left, and it was difficult to process the dead animals and my worry over what was going on with Papa.

That evening the pieces of the puzzle began to fit together in my mind and the story unfolded. Willie was supposed to deliver the groceries to customers who had phoned in their orders that day. The station wagon had been full of groceries when he left with it in the morning, but people started calling in the afternoon to complain that they hadn't received their grocery orders. Willie just disappeared with the station wagon that day. No explanation. Shortly afterwards we found out he had fled to Vancouver.

Things seemed to go back to normal for a short time, but it soon became clear that Papa was under a lot of stress. Normally he was a quiet person when at home, but he began to have some rather serious discussions regarding the store. I never paid much attention until the day I overheard him say with deep emotion, "But I just can't see those kids go hungry!" Papa was in fact struggling to keep the business afloat, but being the kind and generous person he was, he just couldn't say no to the customers who took their groceries on credit. Of course, it was only a matter of time before it finally caught up with him, and, sadly, he lost his business.

He spent a period of time after that going from door to door to collect the money that was owed to him, and he shared a couple of stories with us. At one of the customers' homes, when he knocked on the door a little girl answered. And when he stepped inside, asking to speak with her mother or father, she said they were not at home. But then as he politely responded and turned to leave, he said he caught a slight movement of a curtain off to the side in the living room with a pair of shoes sticking out from underneath. Slightly embarrassed he said he just left without mentioning it.

A new Sears outlet moved into our store's space, and I remember how strange it was to walk past and see the new sign overhead. It became obvious to us how much losing the business affected Papa because once in a while he would walk over and just stand there across the street from the store and stare as if in a trance. I heard Mama on the phone one day saying, "Go and bring your father home!" It embarrassed her that people would see him react in that manner. After a while he did pull himself together. He had no choice but to accept the situation at hand, I suppose, but I do not believe that Papa ever got over the deep disappointment of losing his business on Plummer Avenue. His life had revolved around the store for so many years; it truly was the centre of his life.

As children, of course, we never gave any thought as to what was involved in the closing of the store or how it would affect our lives financially or otherwise. Soon after it was closed, we discovered that some of its contents had been put into storage in our long barn in the field. They managed to find a place in the middle between the horses' stalls and the vehicles, so Anita and I decided to use the long counter from the store as our "stage." We used a large sheet as the curtain. Then we found what looked like a miniature harp with many strings on it, and we would strum on it as if it were a guitar while singing popular songs we'd heard on the radio. We were quite proud to have set up this private little space for ourselves, and we enjoyed being there.

But it wasn't long before someone decided they would have some fun of their own. We came into the barn one day to find our little haven in a complete mess. The curtain was pulled down and all our props were scattered on the floor. We were disappointed, and when I found out it was my nephew Francis, the butcher's son, I confronted him as he came into the yard. My behaviour was—how should I put it?—not very ladylike, as my mother would say. There were no more incidents after that.

Chapter 3

I was aware of only one mine in operation in New Waterford. It was the No. 12 Colliery Mine situated close to our parish of Saint Agnes, which was within walking distance from our school and church. It opened in 1913 and had been in operation for many years. I can still recall the low rumbling sound of the box cars when they began their descent, carrying the miners down into "the pit" as they called it, which ran for a few miles out under the ocean. At noontime, we'd hear the whistle letting everyone know what time of day it was. Then later on—somewhere between eight and nine o'clock if I remember correctly—we'd hear it again, but in a lower tone. It was curfew for the younger ones who might still be outside.

What really stands out in my mind are the miners who lived with the constant danger inherent in their jobs. They seemed to share a sort of unspoken kinship, you might say, most likely due to the fact that they never knew whether they would come out of the pit alive at the end of each shift. Whenever tragic news of yet another miner losing his life came out, the victims' families received tremendous emotional support from the entire town.

A few of my classmates lost their fathers while I was in grade school, and one in particular stands out in my mind. I remember seeing her walking to school shortly after her father's funeral. She was looking straight ahead as if in a world of her own. I felt so sad seeing how pale and drawn she appeared, as if still in shock. And no wonder! To have to live with the thought of the horrific way in which her father had been taken from her. His head was severed in a horrible accident in the mine. Because I didn't know her,

I was too shy to approach and give her my sympathy. But my heart ached for her. Her image haunted me for some time after seeing her that day.

When Papa lost the business on Plummer Avenue, he decided to open another store on a much smaller scale on the outskirts of town. When that did not work out, it was just too much for him to take, I believe. It was around that time, when one day as I was coming in from school through the front door, Papa just happened to be coming out of the living room and into the hallway; he looked rather strange, I thought. Mama was following behind asking him something, and when he did not respond, I saw the concern on her face. He seemed to be incoherent, as if wandering around in deep thought. She took him by the arm, telling him to go upstairs and lie down. That gesture in itself caught my attention because I had never seen her show any concern whatsoever towards him before.

What I did not know was that the doctor had been there just before I arrived. I found out later that when he examined Papa, he suggested Mama call our parish priest to come to the house. She was told he could go into a coma at any moment. Catholics believe that whenever someone is near death, a priest should hear the person's confession so that all their sins would be forgiven. But Papa did not want to speak with him; he wanted to talk with a French priest from another parish because it would be more comfortable to speak in his native tongue. Apparently, Papa's request was granted and he was able to have his confession at home, there in our living room.

The French priest had left just before I came in and found Mama coaxing Papa to go upstairs to rest. He was reluctant but started slowly up the stairs. Mama nudged him along, stopping every so many steps, pausing at the corner landing and finally reaching the hallway. She put him in the spare room across from their bedroom, which I thought was rather odd.

The next day while sitting on the stairway (my spot for observing what was going on around me), I saw Father Campbell standing at the front door talking to Mama. I strained to hear the conversation because they both looked so serious, but they were talking in such low, hushed tones that I was not able to make out anything they were saying. All of a sudden, from upstairs came this spine-chilling scream!

"MA!"

Father Campbell crashed past me up the stairs, taking three steps at a time. My heart pounded as I quickly followed behind. From the top of the stairs, I could see they were in the spare bedroom. Papa was lying on his back looking as if he was asleep. He was covered with a blanket with only his bare feet showing. The priest was standing at the end of the bed holding a book and saying some prayers. Mama was kneeling at the side of the bed next to my sister Adeline. She motioned for me to come in and kneel down with them. We began to say the rosary together.

I suddenly grasped what was actually happening.

"Where is Tony? Go find him," Mama said.

When I went out the back door, I saw that he was down in the field with three of his friends playing baseball. He didn't see me approach because he was at bat and standing over the plate, focused on the pitcher.

"TONY!" I shouted, "Papa just died!"

He flung the bat to the side and we scurried back to the house. As we went through the kitchen, I saw Yvonne on the floor next to the ladder trying to clean up a big blob of white paint that had spilled on the deep blue linoleum floor. She was up on the ladder painting the wall when she heard the scream coming from upstairs and panicked.

Adeline told us that Papa had asked her to help him to the bathroom. While she was helping him get back into bed, she said he suddenly swerved sideways and she wasn't able to grasp him. His eyes rolled up and she screamed.

Amidst all the commotion, Anita and I retreated to the back porch in disbelief that our Papa had suddenly passed away. We were standing in the corner holding onto each other when the door opened and in walked Junior, who was a sergeant major in the army. He had just flown in from out west where he was stationed. As he put his luggage down, he said in a derogatory tone, "Oh stop your snivelling." We were startled but not really surprised because he always made belittling remarks.

Papa was laid out in our living room in front of the double windows, so I had a glimpse of him through the French doors. They opened the top part of the casket and I could see his head, but I was afraid to go into the room. I stood there peering through the glass squares of the French doors at Adeline. She reached over and stroked his forehead saying, "He's so cold." I turned and ran upstairs to lie down on the bed where Papa was when he passed away. I closed my eyes for a few moments, and when I opened them, my mind suddenly froze when I saw a hand—someone else's hand?—resting on the pillow in front of me.

I jumped up and ran downstairs past the living room, but I was afraid to look in as I passed the door. When I told Mama about the hand, she must have realized that I was having a difficult time because Anita and I were taken to Aunt Lena's house. Papa's sister lived in a big, beautiful white house a few minutes' drive away. It was the first time we had been in their home, and we were told we would spend a few days there. Our cousin Dolly, a nurse, lived there and took time off work the next day to take the two of us out for ice cream. She really tried to make us feel welcome, but I was too shy because of all the unexpected attention we were given. I just remember feeling embarrassed whenever they tried to talk to us.

Besides Anita and I living at home, there was Tony (two years older than us), Yvonne (sixteen), Justine and Adeline. Some of our older brothers and sisters had been placed in boarding schools at an early age, and Justine was one of them. After the funeral, it was decided that a photographer should come in to take a family photo. When I saw the pictures later, I noticed that not everyone was present. They were not able to find my brother Willie—the one who had left for Vancouver with all the groceries—to give him the bad news. So we were surprised when he showed up a couple of years after Papa's passing. He was shocked to learn of Papa's death and was ashamed not to have stayed in touch with the family. He was a quiet, rather passive person who was very gentle with our cat. Unfortunately, he began to take comfort in the bottle before he left, and he drifted even further away from the family over time.

I never had much interest in school, especially after Papa died, and I often made excuses not to go. One day Anita must have come up with a better excuse than mine, or maybe she really was not well, but for whatever reason I ended up walking home from school all alone. I was so used to having her with me all the time that I felt empty, and the feeling gradually worsened as I got closer to home.

Feeling totally disconnected from the world, I was about to cross the street. I checked to see if any cars were coming when this horrible thought passed through my mind: *What would happen if I just stepped out in front of that big truck that is coming my way?* As it passed by in front of me, I continued my slow walk homeward. Thoughts like, *Nobody would come to my funeral anyway* circled in my mind. I had this deep conviction that I truly did not belong in this world; that's how worthless I felt.

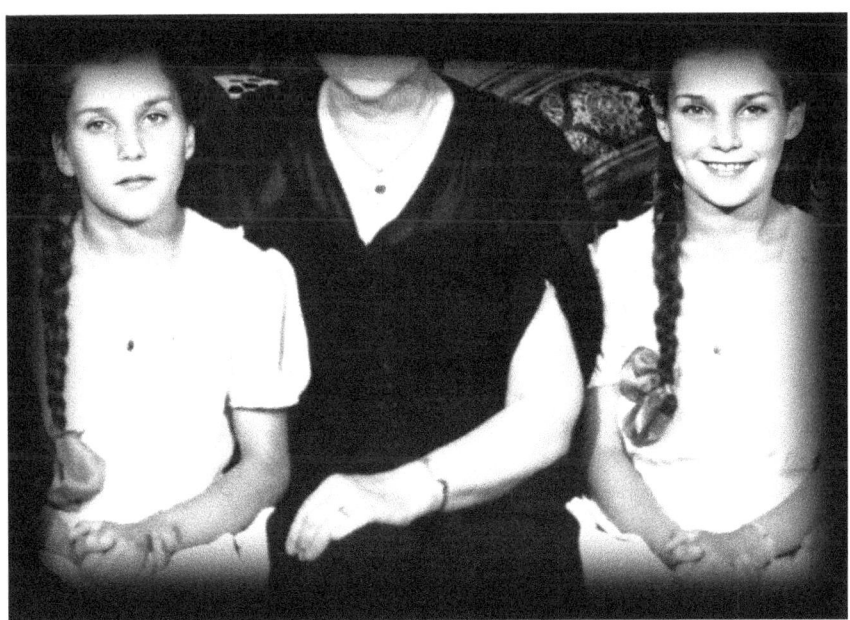

Anna and Anita, 9 years old

I didn't realize it showed until I came into the house.

"You were walking with slumped shoulders," Mama said, "Why don't you straighten up!"

I didn't say anything because I knew that any emotional needs would be quickly brushed aside. We all learned from an early age that we could never turn to her for any kind of support or understanding. As a matter of fact, Anita and I had agreed just a few days before that it was Mama who should have been taken from us—not Papa! We wished someone would come along and adopt us because we knew that Mama felt stuck with us. She was just waiting for a time when she could finally get rid of us altogether.

The emotional pain just got worse with each passing day.

After Papa died, Mama received what was called a "Widow's Allowance," but it was not sufficient because I remember coming home from school many times when there was hardly anything to eat. If we were lucky, we'd find a crust of bread at the bottom of the big, round, silver bread box on the pantry floor where there had always been fresh loaves of home-made bread in the past.

I was so hungry that I began to have bad headaches quite often and was not able to see clearly; it was sort of like seeing spots in front of me. During one of our home economics classes at school, the sister who was teaching held up a saucer with half a grapefruit on it with a cherry on top. She was telling us that whoever had a number to match the one she was about to pick would win the prize—a grapefruit. Nothing special, I know, but my mouth watered as I sent up a little prayer, *Please let it be for me.* But another classmate had the matching number. When she put it down in front of her and began talking to the others as if she didn't even want it, I thought, *She has no idea how much I want to have that piece of grapefruit.*

No one realized how desperate the situation at home was after Papa's passing. We were always well dressed in clothes that Mama ordered from the thick Sears and Eaton's catalogues we had in those days. When an older brother, Jimmy, came home from Montreal for a short visit, I heard him say to Mama, "Why don't you go and get welfare?"

"Oh Jimmy, they're not going to *believe* that the Ouellettes have no money!" she said.

But as time passed, it started to show outwardly that Anita and I were not eating properly. Slowly but surely, we were losing weight and losing interest in everything else. Another brother, Joseph, came home from either Montreal or Toronto to visit not long after Jimmy returned to Montreal. He tried to help by stealing a huge bag of potatoes from U Get More to make French fries. However, when Mama learned that he didn't pay for the potatoes, she insisted that he take them back immediately!

Not long after that, Anita and I were sitting outside on the back step on a warm, sunny day. The kitchen windows next to the step were open and we could hear Mama and my sister Justine (who had recently married George, a neighbour of ours) talking. Our ears opened with curiosity when we heard the word "twins" mentioned, so we crept down the few steps to get under the kitchen window and listen intently. It became clear that she was selling our house to Justine and George, but Mama would also stay living with us. When we heard Justine say, "I'll take the twins," we glanced at each other in wide-eyed anticipation. Could this really be happening? Then she added, "They can stay until they turn eighteen."

Aside from getting our bits and pieces of information at home in this manner, we really had no way of knowing what was happening around us. And with the understanding from a very early age that we were to be seen but not heard, I guess we knew better than to pester with questions. We both became very anxious because we never heard anything more about selling the house, so finally I asked Mama, "Will Justine be coming to visit us again?" She had no idea that Anita and I had overheard that conversation regarding selling our house.

"No she's not feeling well," Mama said. "She's been having bad migraine headaches lately."

This kinda left us just hanging, so to speak, with no clue as to what would become of our situation.

Shortly after that, however, Mama told us that Justine had to go into the hospital in New Waterford. The next day we heard that she went unconscious and had to be taken to the St. Edward Hospital outside of New Waterford. They discovered she had tuberculosis (TB). She had only been married six months, so we were shocked when told she was not expected to live.

She remained unconscious for two weeks when the wonderful news that she had regained consciousness came to us! When she was finally allowed visitors, only the adults in the family could go in. Even so, someone managed to sneak Anita and me in because Justine had asked to see us. I was very surprised when I saw her. She was sitting up and smiling but looked so different. Before she went into the hospital, she was very thin and pale, even in her wedding picture. But now her face was chubby and she had rosy cheeks. We could only have a few minutes while standing at the doorway, then were smuggled out again. Her devoted husband George was at her side constantly. They joked that his car would soon be able to find its own way to the hospital.

Justine spent a few months in the St. Edward's Annex before she and George went to live with his parents a couple of houses down from our place. The doctor said that even though she survived, she would never be the same. I did not understand what he meant, but we began to slowly realize what he was trying to tell us.

After Tony went to find work in Montreal, there was just Anita and I left at home with Mama. I started to have difficulty with math in Grade 5; I simply could not understand what some of the questions meant or how to solve the problems; it was terribly frustrating. I hated school by then and didn't want to go anymore. Whenever I muttered this under my breath, Mama would say, "You have to go! At least till Grade 9!"

We were transferred from our old school, which was a two-storey building, into the new high school that was built just behind it. It was a long building with only one floor, and it had a large gym at one end. Anita and I rarely opened our books to do any homework at all that year, and consequently we both ended up having to repeat the sixth grade.

That was the year we had a new teacher who drove in from Glace Bay, which was about ten minutes away. The students did not like him at all, and they began to call him Ichabod Crane. He had a mean spirit and he actually seemed to pick on some of the students. During class one morning, he asked a question regarding something he had just read to us. I often refrained from putting my hand up to answer questions because I was afraid I would say the wrong answer. But more often than not, when a student put their hand up and had the wrong answer, I'd say to myself, *I should have put my hand up! I knew the answer to that question!* Anyway, he was writing something on the chalkboard, and he turned to ask what about the difference between such and such—something he had just finished explaining. I wasn't quite sure if I had the correct answer this time, but I shot my hand up anyway. When I answered and it was incorrect, I did not like the way he swiftly and sternly replied "NO," gesturing for me to sit down as he quickly pointed to another student for an answer.

This belittling attitude along with his negative energy stirred a reaction within me that not only surprised him and the rest of the class, but also caught me by surprise too. As he shot the other person down in the same manner when the wrong answer was given, I deliberately stood there next to my desk and glared at him defiantly. He gestured again with a wave of dismissal and said in a derogatory tone, "Sit down!" In that moment I decided to simply refuse to obey his command. For a second, he appeared as if he did not know what to do with me, then in total frustration he turned and bolted out the door. I stood there steadfast, determined I was not going to budge.

Amidst the high tension in the room, I could see the class was actually on my side. Moments later, he reappeared with the principal, who happened to be a nun, following behind. She looked rather impatient and annoyed. Some of the students were giggling, and I could hear nervous whispers just behind me.

"SIT DOWN, Miss Ouellette!" he said loudly and sternly.

When I refused again, the room fell silent. The principal motioned for me to follow her out of the room. As we walked down the hallway to her office, I was still feeling defiant. She told me to sit down in front of her desk, so I was expecting some kind of punishment for my behaviour. Instead, she calmly asked what happened to make him so upset. When I explained that I refused to be treated that way and decided to remain standing in protest, I was rather surprised that she responded with a nod as if to say, "I understand."

The recess bell rang, and I felt a wave of relief when she told me that it was okay for me to leave. As I did, the students were pouring out of their classrooms into the hallway. One of them happened to see me, and I was very surprised when he rushed over to me with a big grin on his face.

"You got him real good!" he said.

I must admit that it did give a little boost to my confidence that day. It made me think it was okay to stand up to him the way I did, even though I knew Mama would definitely not have approved!

Chapter 4

Not long after that incident at school, Father Campbell invited Anita and I to go ice skating at the arena in Sydney, a fifteen minute drive from New Waterford. I wasn't interested, but since Anita was, I went along. There were three other girls from our school with us that day. After piling into the long black car, he proudly demonstrated how the windows rolled up and down with the press of a button. It definitely was not as common a feature as it is today, and, of course, we were impressed. A couple of them had gone to the arena with him before, but this was the first time Anita and I went.

It was a rather foggy day with heavy mist in the air. As we approached Sydney, we had to drive through an area called Whitney Pier, where there was a large steel mill. When we slowed down at a railroad crossing, one of the girls said, "Pee-ew! What is that awful smell?" What happened next was something I would never have expected to hear from anyone I knew, let alone from our parish priest. Without blinking an eye he chuckled, "They're burning n----- babies." I was stunned and astonished that they actually thought he was being funny. A revealing moment indeed.

Anita and I were woken up one morning by a loud noise just outside our bedroom window. When I opened the venetian blind, I was surprised to see a huge tractor digging a hole in the field not far from our house. We had not heard anything about what it might be, so we were curious as to what was going on.

Father Campbell had been coming to visit Mama on a regular basis, and a lawyer from Sydney had come to our home a number of times as well. I'd see this bald, rather chubby man with glasses perched near the tip of his nose sitting at our dining-room table, focused on a bunch of papers spread out in front of him. This was shortly after Papa's funeral, at a time when Mama was in a vulnerable state of mind. In retrospect, it is obvious what the priest had in mind. He managed to persuade Mama to donate the field next to our house to the parish. Before Mama was able to even think straight, our long barn was taken down and work was underway to build a large, modern ice-skating rink.

The entire field was gradually transformed from Mahon Street, where our house was situated, all the way over to Saint-Anne Street. Long, thin pipes were laid on the ground, welded together and covered with cement. Then a small building was made from large grey blocks at one end of the field; it contained the ammonia needed to freeze the artificial ice. The project was finally completed with a parking lot next to the entrance in the back.

As you came inside the building, the wicket and canteen were on the right side of a large room with varnished wood on the walls and thick wooden benches all along the sides. In the centre stood a black potbelly stove that everyone loved. It kept the place toasty warm for when they'd come in for little breaks during skating time. On the outside facing the rink was a sheltered area with benches and a swinging gate where you'd step onto the ice. The entire rink had a wall with a chain-link fence all along the top, and the whole area was lit with bright lights on high poles that also held the loud speakers. They played beautiful music to skate to that could not only be heard around the rink, but up to the main street of Plummer Ave and beyond. I can still hear the music playing and remember how much we enjoyed skating there.

Father Campbell was somewhat of a star back then as he almost always had some lady on his arm who was obviously the best skater around. We were impressed to see how they waltzed around the ice. I must admit I did like the attention when, once in a while, he'd come alongside and grab my hand to go a few rounds with him. We didn't waltz, though; that was only with a couple of the best skaters. He'd have one arm around her waist and the other one holding her hand up in the waltz position. While skating backwards he skilfully and smoothly guided her along. This would take place the night after the hockey games, when the ice was at it's best because it had been groomed with the Zamboni. It had brushes that turned underneath as it slowly moved along while watering the ice; the result was like a clear sheet of glass. Anita and I were actually pretty good skaters, but I can't say the same for roller skating, which was what it was used for during the summertime. I think Anita and I only gave it a few tries before we decided it was not for us.

Just before Justine and George bought our house, Mama had arranged for Anita and I to go to Dartmouth near Halifax to stay with our oldest sister Inez. She lived with her husband, who worked for an oil company there, and their three boys. We knew this was one of Mama's last attempts to get rid of us. She had arranged for our brother Frankie, who used to work as the butcher when we had our store, to drive us since he made regular trips to Halifax while working for the *Halifax Herald* after Papa died. He reluctantly agreed to take us to Inez's place in the truck he used on those trips, but I really did not like the idea of going on that trip with him. He was the one who had threatened to bury me in a hole that he was digging when I was a little child, and I was terrified of him. So it was very uncomfortable to have to spend hours with him knowing he really did not want to take us; we both knew what a bother we were for him. After driving for quite some time, I noted it was midnight when we finally stopped at a rooming house along the way. In the morning, we continued on to my sister's place in Dartmouth.

When we arrived, I found Inez to be a little distant with us, but she was at least receptive when she opened the door. That same day she suggested we go to the store and buy a tub of ice cream, "To put some meat on your bones." Strange how the mind works sometimes, because as I'm writing this sentence, a memory just flashed of myself walking past a restaurant (in the back where some food had been thrown out) where I spotted an orange peel that had spilled out of a bag that was lying on the ground. I remember I was so hungry I walked over, picked it up and ate the rind inside the orange peeling.

Anyway, back to Inez's place.

After the two weeks were up, Inez told us that Frankie would come by to take us back to Cape Breton. So we had to return to the same situation where we went without proper meals, and the never-ending feeling of not being wanted. I believe we were thirteen, maybe fourteen years old at that time.

On our regular walks to school, Anita and I often passed by the little bungalow where Justine and George lived with his parents. Sometimes when George's father happened to be sitting outside on the step, he'd motion for us to come over. He would simply smile as he handed each of us a quarter. We were very shy, so we just thanked him then went home to show Mama.

"Go to the corner store down the road and buy a quart of milk and a package of fig newtons with that money," she would say.

For anyone else this would have been a nice little treat. But it was much more for Anita and me. We hadn't enough to eat in the few years since Papa had died, so it almost felt like a meal. We were grateful for his kindness. So when we heard that George's father had suddenly passed away, we were surprised and felt sad because he was such a loving person. Apparently when he got up to go to work as usual and was preparing his lunch to take to work with him, he suddenly collapsed on the kitchen floor from a heart attack. We often thought about him as we passed by after that, remembering what a kind and gentle person he was.

Anita and I seemed to change and grow at a much slower pace than everyone else. I also couldn't help but notice how our classmates were moving forward with their lives and were occupied with things they were interested in and excited about. They were open to making new friends, for example, while we remained distant—even childlike.

As far back as I can remember, we had braids in our hair, but after Justine and George moved in with us, Mama allowed us to have them cut off. You'd think I would remember the first time we had our braids cut off, but I don't; I just know I did not like the way I looked afterwards. Not long after that, Mama let us get our hair done at the hairdresser where she went on a regular basis to get a perm. Her hair turned white rather early in life, so she began to have the light bluish tinge added like some others had at that time. Anita and I had our first perm in a style that had the flat waves on top with tight curls around the bottom. It was quite popular, and the change was noticeable, because we had many comments from our classmates at school.

This brings to mind someone I did not know very well but would often see delivering the newspaper along our street. His name was Mike. I also saw him at church since he was an altar boy there. He was probably a couple of years younger than us. Anyway, at our school each class had to form a line before going into the building. One day soon after we'd had our hair done, Mike was holding the door open for the classes to go inside, and I couldn't help but notice him staring at Anita and I. When we passed in front of him, we were close enough that I could see his big brown eyes, and I was startled when he actually winked at me. I thought, *Oh, he's so cute!* I knew that he had a crush on the both of us which lasted for quite a while, but we never did get to speak to him other than a "Hi" now and then because all three of us were too shy to actually talk to one another.

Around that time, changes started to take place at home when Justine and George decided to buy our house. Everyone agreed that the three of us—Anita, Mama and I—would live there until we turned eighteen. Mama wanted to sell the house because she was not able keep it financially and feed us at the same time. She managed to hang onto it for three years after Papa died, but Anita and I slowly became very thin from malnutrition. Besides that, the deep feelings of the years of emotional and mental neglect began to surface.

I was painfully aware of how other classmates had much more self-esteem than Anita and me. They functioned so well and seemed confident. My self-image was always low to begin with, and by then I had no sense of self-worth whatsoever.

So when Justine and George moved in, I found the change was for the better, giving me a glimmer of hope. At least we had food on the table when we came home from school, and we were pleasantly surprised when Justine bought each of us a wristwatch and a medallion with a mirror on one side. This attention from her, along with our new hair do, gave a little boost to our morale.

There was some talk at home regarding adoption. I understood that Justine and George had their name on a list to adopt a baby, but we never thought much about it; we were more focused on starting this new phase of our lives, I suppose. And, of course, after the move, we all had to make some adjustments. In the beginning, we had no problem getting used to the little changes like Justine being very conscious of cleanliness. Our place wasn't untidy before, it was fine, but now there was a place for everything and everything had its place, so to speak. And we were to follow this new system exactly.

I never went through a stage of teenage rebellion. In fact, I can only recall that one incident at school with the nun where I stepped out of line. One time—I was probably eight or nine years old—when I felt frustrated with Mama and muttered under my breath, "Oh shut up." I was instantly slapped across the face, and she said, "You don't talk to your mother like that!" Otherwise, I can honestly say that I always tried to do as I was told. I actually believed it was a sin to disobey your parents. I even told the priest (during confessional time at church) that I had disobeyed my mother, and I was given a penance there in the little cubicle where we went to confess our sins.

For those wanting to go to confession, there was a special place in the church right next to the pews where you'd step into this small boxlike area in the wall and close the door behind you. There was a little screened window on the wall where the priest sat on the other side, but we couldn't see each other. He'd ask us what we had to confess, then we were given a penance—usually to say a couple of prayers or maybe a few beads of the rosary—then our so-called sins would be forgiven. I actually didn't have any problem with this since it made us stop, think and examine our conscience. It actually felt good to believe that we were forgiven for whatever wrong we did.

When Justine took over, I don't recall having any problems adjusting to our new situation, I just felt that our lives were more structured than before. I missed the little things, though, like being able to play our games of Chinese checkers, Snakes and Ladders, Monopoly, etc. that we used to play on our big, round oak table in the dining room. Our nephews, who were Frankie the butcher's children, lived just behind our house and would come in to play the games with us once in a while. But that table was removed when Justine moved in, along with the radio and pull-out record player on the bottom that held the large 78-speed records. It was replaced with a new television set. We were okay with that because it was what Justine wanted and it was her house now after all.

Anita and I had gained a couple of pounds and were starting to feel a little better about ourselves in general. But as time passed, I began to understand what that doctor meant when said that Justine would never be the same after surviving TB. She slowly started to show that she was not comfortable with us being there anymore. There were never arguments or raised voices, just uneasy feelings that I can recall.

Like the time at the dinner table when I reached for something and accidentally knocked over my glass of milk. She quickly removed the white tablecloth and said in a low, impatient tone, "George, either they go, or I go." If I forgot to hang my uniform up on a hanger when I got home from school, she would get upset. I remember we had to sit in the dining room and watch television while she prepared supper because she preferred to do everything herself, and we didn't have the simple freedom to just move around the house and do whatever we felt like doing. It was rather difficult to deal with at times.

She meant well and was actually a very kind person who did the best she knew how. She could not help it that her mental health was affected by that terrible disease. The fact that she survived was a miracle in itself. It was obvious that George loved and respected her very much and, being grateful that she had recovered, he always tried to help with a caring and loving attitude.

Chapter 5

In our second year living with Justine and George, they rented a tiny cabin on a beach in Mira Gut for the summer. They came out for short visits on Sundays while Anita and I stayed there with Mama for the whole summer. For whatever reason, Mama did not like to be on the beach herself, which was only yards away from the cabin. She preferred to stay inside while the two of us spent most of our time in the water enjoying our very first vacation there at Mira Gut.

From inside the cabin I could hear the soothing sounds of little waves rolling onto the beach with it's constant rhythmic motion, and I loved the calming effect it had on my mind as I fell asleep at night. The setting sun always brought a change in both energy and scenery alike, and one evening in particular comes to mind. We were about to leave for the large recreation hall, which was a ten-minute walk from the cabin, where they had a jukebox and dancing in the evenings. As Anita and I stepped out onto the unpaved road in front our cabin, we caught the last rays of the sun as it slowly disappeared. In those few moments of quiet stillness, with the crimson colour reflecting on the water, I had this incredibly peaceful feeling of oneness with nature. It was a spiritual type of connection where I was filled with gratitude just to experience those beautifully simple moments. As we started to walk slowly along the side of the road, we could hear the soothing voice of Dean Martin singing "Return to Me" floating across the countryside and adding a touch of sweetness to the evening air.

Our pace picked up with anticipation of what was waiting for us. Firewood for a bonfire was ready to go, and there would be a corn boil that evening on the beach. The music drew us inside even though only a handful of people had arrived by then. This was our first time there, but it didn't take long before we were moving on the dance floor to what was called the "jive." Anita and I only danced with each other and we made up the steps as we went along. We really enjoyed listening and dancing to the "rock 'n' roll" music. By the end of that summer, we took those happy memories home with us.

Between the time when we arrived back home from our summer vacation, and just before school opened in the fall, Anita and I took little walks along the main street of Plummer Avenue for the first time. We were about sixteen years old. We'd sit on a bench in the park next to a statue that was there in memory of the miners who had lost their lives. That's where we met a guy who's nickname was Beanie. He walked around with a little brown cloth beanie on his head that had tiny holes in it. He liked to point out the names of the cars as they passed by and the year they were made. The next time when we were there we'd try to remember.

On one nice sunny Sunday afternoon while we were sitting there on the bench, this white horse came prancing along the main street in front of us. I remember the sound of its hooves clip-clopping on the pavement and its thick tail softly flowing behind. The rider rode bareback, looking straight ahead as if he were in some kind of a parade. I couldn't help but notice two large letters—US—that were seared into the horse's rump. I was curious and would have liked to have a chance to speak with him, but he was gone as quickly as he had appeared.

Not long after that Sunday afternoon, Anita and I were at Adeline's house on the highway just outside of town. We didn't go there very often, and the few times we did it was to go for a swim in the "channel," as it was called. It was still warm enough to get another swim in before the summer came to a close, so we crossed the highway in front of her house and then walked a couple of minutes through the bush to the water. As we came to the opening at the end of the path, we were surprised to see what looked like the same horse we had seen in town a few weeks ago. It was standing at the water's edge nibbling on some grass, and someone was sitting on the ground holding the reins.

I had this strong urge to go over and talk to him, and as I approached, I saw that it was the same person and same horse. When I asked if I could pet the horse, he half smiled and nodded. I started the conversation by telling him about us sitting in the park that day we happened to see him riding down the main street in town. I said I'd noticed the letters and wanted to know what they meant. He said the horse was used in the military in the United States but was now retired.

As I was gently stroking the horse's nose, he asked, "Do you want to go for a ride?" Anita answered yes before I had a chance to respond, so I was obviously annoyed with her as he helped her climb up onto the horse's back.

"He asked me, not you!" I said.

But after a short ride around the immediate area next to the water, he helped her down then turned to me and asked again, "Do you want to go for a ride?"

"Yes, I would love to," I said.

He bent down and cupped his hands together for me to step in so I could climb up. He then sat behind me and, taking the reins gently, nudged the horse to start walking.

His name was Dougie, he said, and the horse's name was Bob. A couple of minutes later, we reached the paved highway and continued on from there. About ten minutes later we turned off to our right onto a long gravel road, and as we slowly moved along Lingan Road, as it was called, I felt the need to stop and rest a bit. So when I spotted a large log on the side of the road, I pointed to it and asked if we could sit and rest on that for a while. He agreed, and we made some small talk. I could tell he was proud of Bob and that he was quite confident in the way he was handling him.

I sat there watching as he got back up on the horse and started giving him instructions to move backwards. He firmly pulled upwards on the reins and the horse suddenly reared up on his hind legs and came down again. Wow! I loved it.

I started to wonder about the ride back to Adeline's place because I had some cramps and my rear end was hurting by then. He suggested we go to his sister's place about a half mile away. I was glad to hear about that, so we decided to keep going until we reached Roaches Road, which turned out to be where Dougie lived.

He passed by his house and continued on through a field that took us to where his sister lived. She happened to be outside and looked surprised to see us come strolling by. A rather heavyset person, she seemed friendly enough when Dougie introduced us. Her name was Olga. When she saw I was having trouble trying to walk properly after I slid down from the horse, she invited us to go inside. My first impression was that they were a close-knit family. Before too long, it was decided that I should be driven home, which I was very thankful for.

When I finally got home, it was supper time and I remembered we had left Anita at the channel. I consoled myself by thinking she simply had to walk a few minutes to get back to Adeline's place and would be just fine.

When I went upstairs to freshen up before supper, I noticed a spot of blood on my underwear. I figured it must be the beginning of a period, since I had not started to menstruate yet. Turned out it was not that after all, and when I finally did get my first period, I was much older than most girls. Later on, I realized that since I had never been intimate with anyone (I was a virgin) that riding without a saddle caused the hymen to break, resulting in the discomfort and spotting of blood.

About a week or so after that first ride on Bob the horse, I was surprised when Dougie showed up outside our house. Apparently he had walked by just to see where we lived. While Anita and I were outside chatting with him, we asked if he'd like to have supper with us. I don't think he was comfortable because he did not want to stay very long. We did meet up again at the Chinese restaurant in town that had a jukebox with all the hit tunes of the fifties that I really liked. I got the impression that this was a place where Dougie liked to hang out with another friend who was there with him that day.

Shortly after that, as Anita and I were walking past a little bungalow on the other side of town, we stopped to talk with a new friend we had met recently. She was about our age with an outgoing happy type of personality. She seemed to like us, and she invited us to a party at her house that weekend. We asked Mama, but both her and Justine didn't like the idea at first. I was happy when they suddenly gave in and we were allowed to go.

Because we never had parties in our house, I didn't know what to expect when we got there. I hoped there would be some dancing, which we were excited about. We really liked the rock 'n' roll music they played, and we were able to show off our new jive moves that we'd picked up that summer in Mira Gut. Before too long, the small living room became quite crowded. I was surprised to see Dougie come in and sit there on the sidelines with a beer in his hand. He didn't get up to dance, so I sat down with him for a while, but before I knew it, I was right back up on the floor again when Anita tugged at me to get up and dance with her. We were so caught up in the music that we paid no attention whatsoever to what time it was. When someone mentioned that it was after eleven thirty, it jolted our minds because we had promised we would not stay out too late. I pulled Anita to the side and said, "We have to leave now!" When we left through the front door just off the living room, we could still hear the music as we stepped out onto the road.

"We shouldn't have stayed out so long," I said. "Mama is going to be mad at us!"

"I know!" said Anita.

Both of us were afraid of what we would face when we got home. She reminded me of what had happened just a few weeks ago when we were on our way home from Mary's house (our best friend). It was the only time we had ever been allowed out late at night. Beanie and his buddy just happened to be standing at the corner of Plummer Avenue and our street where we had to pass directly in front of them. As we did, Beanie made a silly joke that made us laugh, and before we knew it, we were talking back and forth without giving any thought as to what time it was. There was a quiet peacefulness in the deserted streets that night as we stood there chatting when a determined-looking figure came walking along Mahon Street in our direction. We fell silent, straining to see who this person might be.

"Oh my God," I whispered. "It's Mama!"

"Oh no!" said Beanie, as he spun around on his heel to face the building, as if trying to hide his face from her.

She quickly grabbed Anita and I by the scruffs of our necks, and while shoving us in front of her muttered, "Standing on the street corner talking to boys at this hour of the night!"

To say we were embarrassed is an understatement; we were humiliated!

So as Anita and I walked home from the party with that memory still fresh in our minds, we could only anticipate the worst would be waiting for us when we got home.

As we entered our yard, the house was in complete darkness, so we went around to the back porch hoping we'd get in through the back door. It was locked. We then gingerly crept up onto the veranda and tried to open the front door—nope, it, too, was locked! We just stared at each other not knowing what to do.

We slid down and sat on the floor of the veranda. She suggested maybe we should walk out to Adeline's place, even though it was a few miles away. I agreed we had to do something, so we walked up the hill and crossed Plummer Avenue. From there we quickly walked along the sidewalk until we reached Scotch Town, which is a part of New Waterford, where the houses became farther apart as the road turned into a highway.

While walking along on the left side of the road facing traffic, I was startled when what looked like an animal about the size of a cat suddenly dashed across the highway in front of us. Even though it was dark I was able to see the image. Each time a vehicle came by, the bright lights began to bother me. One time a car slowed down and followed us for a short distance before it sped away. We were nervous, so from then on whenever we saw on-coming bright lights, we crouched down in the wide ditch along the highway.

We were pretty tired by the time we reached Adeline's place and were not surprised when we saw that the house was in total darkness. I had no idea how long we were walking, I just knew it was very late by the time we had reached the small back step. We sat down, wondering what to do next.

Anita asked, "Should we knock on the door?"

"No, it's too late! We'll have to stay here on the step until morning."

We were sitting up with our backs against the wall, and I remember dozing off and feeling very cold. At one point, I was tempted to knock on the door but was held back by the fear of how they would react when they found us.

When morning finally arrived, I awoke with warm rays of sunlight on my face. I could barely open my eyes, feeling stiff and sore all over. The black colour of my pants drew the sun's rays through the material, which felt good and made me want to stay there absorbing the much-needed heat. I turned to see Anita next to me. She was still asleep, so I nudged her gently.

"Wake up, it's morning," I said. "We have to let them know we're here."

She squinted, slowly looked around and said, "Oh no, this is not a dream—it's for real!"

"Yes, so I'm going to knock on the door now, okay?"

At that very moment, the door opened quickly and Adeline was standing there in her housecoat, an angry, baffled look on her face.

"How did you get here?" she exclaimed.

I tried to say something, but she leaned inside the doorway and shouted, "The twins are out here on the step! Come inside. I'm going to call Justine."

We timidly followed her into the house where she went directly to the phone and dialed home. She was clearly frustrated with us and we knew we were in big trouble. I was feeling more anxious by the minute.

"Justine just told me that they will come to get you," she said as she hung up the phone.

I explained that we had left the party as soon as we realized what time it was, but when we got home the doors were locked. I said we didn't know what to do, so we came here.

"But how did you get here?" she demanded.

"We walked," I said.

By now I was so exhausted physically, mentally and emotionally that I must have shut down because I do not remember anything after that. Not even when they came to pick us up, let alone when we finally reached home that morning. The last thing I recall is staring at Adeline, who was demanding to know what was going on, when a terrifying image came into in my mind. It was of me in a small, dark room desperately trying to keep a heavy steel door open that was slowly closing in on me inch by inch. Then my mind actually went blank.

Because no one said a word the next day about our being locked out and ending up on Adeline's step all night, I never knew what they were thinking. Many years later when I called Mama, which was about the only time I spoke to her over the phone (there never was any kind of dialogue between us, ever), I asked why they locked us out that night. She said that they drove around a few streets looking for us, but when they couldn't find us, they must have locked the door. Then she said something that surprised me.

"When you came in the next morning you looked very strange. When we asked questions you suddenly became hysterical. I had never seen you act like that before."

Hearing that, at least I had an inkling as to what might have happened to me mentally and emotionally that night we were locked out. I must have been overwhelmed by the whole experience and most likely had some sort of a mental breakdown.

Unfortunately, this turned out to be just the beginning of similar episodes throughout my life whenever I felt helpless or rejected. To this day, I still have unanswered questions about that night. Maybe they left us there for a while as a form of punishment—to teach us a lesson but with the intention of opening the door at some point? Guess I'll never know. But I've learned that if there is no way to express one's feelings openly and honestly regarding something that affected us in a negative way during those impressionable years, it doesn't just go away. It stays with us and affects how we react to situations later on in life.

Chapter 6

Back at school in the fall, Anita and I were puzzled when Father Campbell came to the high school one day to have a talk with us. When he asked how we were getting along at home, I guess it was apparent that we were not doing all that well. Before he ended the discussion, he asked, "Would you like to move in with a family that lives only five minutes away from where you are living on Mahon Street?"

He went on to explain that there was a family who owned the jewellery store on Plummer Avenue. The father had passed away, and now there was just the mother living there with her two children who were a little younger than Anita and me. I knew who he was talking about because I'd seen them in church on Sundays but never actually spoken to them.

By then, Dougie had started to work in the mines. He was seventeen years old and bought his first vehicle, a second-hand Ford. It started by pushing a button on the dashboard, and the gear shift was on the steering column. It wasn't very long before I was steering it as we drove along Lingan Road, a gravel road on the outskirts of New Waterford where Dougie lived. Eventually he let me get behind the wheel and I'd drive for about a mile or so before he took over. Once in a while, Dougie would show up when Anita and I were coming home from school. He'd pull up alongside of us and ask if we'd like a lift home. I considered him to be my boyfriend by then, because we saw each other almost every weekend.

Anita didn't have a so-called steady boyfriend, but there was a guy named Winston would come by and take her out for a drive once in a while. He had a dark blue late-model car, and he was a nice, respectful person whom

Anita and I felt was trustworthy. One Sunday when he came by for Anita, he asked me if I would like to go along with them for a drive out on the highway. It was a beautiful sunny evening, and I was happy to be invited because Dougie was at home that weekend helping his brothers Hartigan and Ewen. His family owned three racehorses, and during what they called the haying season they had to be out in the field with a machine cutting the grass. It was then left to dry and subsequently made into bundles of hay for the horses to eat during the winter.

On the highway, we saw a pale green car that looked exactly like Dougie's in front of us.

Winston said, "I think that's Dougie's car in front."

As he got closer to get a better look, the green car slowed down, signalling it was about to make a left turn. As it turned the corner, I blurted out, "Yes, that's him! That's Dougie!" I was shocked to see another girl sitting very close to him.

"And he just turned into the drive-in theatre!" Anita said.

She was just as surprised as I was. For a brief moment we just stared at each other—we were speechless. Winston slowly picked up speed and we continued our drive. They obviously felt sorry for me, so Anita asked if I wanted to go home.

I didn't want to be around anybody when we got back, so I just went to my room and laid there, numb, for quite a long time before a few tears appeared. Strangely enough, I can't remember shedding any tears in my childhood except for a few the day our Papa passed away. But even then, I didn't feel the deep emotional grief I'd seen other people display when their loved ones departed. There were times when I questioned whether I actually had feelings of so-called "love."

But that changed when I met Dougie.

He was the first and only person I ever got close to, so I became emotionally attached. In my innocence, I believed he loved me and that we would always be together. I was left totally confused. After lying awake for most of the night, I finally fell asleep.

The next morning as Anita and I walked to school, the silence between us was a little strange. It was different than just our usual not having anything to say. We never did have normal conversations like most siblings do because we sort of knew what was going on in each other's minds. That Monday morning, though, I felt a bit of apprehension because neither one of us seemed to know how to express in words what was spinning around in our heads regarding the night before. So we just quietly walked along amidst the uncertainty. We just didn't how to react to the situation.

On our way home, we were caught off guard when Dougie casually pulled up alongside of us as he usually did, leaned over and rolled down the passenger-side window.

"Want a ride home?"

Anita stopped and glanced at me wondering if I'd accept, but I didn't respond. I just kept walking ahead without saying a word. Dougie drove very slowly alongside of us and then stopped for a moment and leaned over to open the passenger-side door.

"Come on, get in!" he said.

When I continued walking with my head held high, suppressing my emotions, he finally stopped. This time he opened his door and said, "What's wrong?"

But I felt deeply hurt and just wanted him to go away.

"Why don't you get in and talk to him," Anita said. "I'll walk the rest of the way home."

I hesitated for a moment, then got in. But I sat with my head turned away, looking out the window to my right.

"Are you mad at me?" he asked, looking so innocent.

I couldn't hold back any longer, so I said, "I'd like to know what you were doing yesterday around supper time."

"I had to help my brother with the haying like I said, why?"

Being the Sagittarius I am, I pulled out my bow and arrow and aimed my question straight at him.

"Who were you with when you went to the drive-in theatre yesterday?"

"What? What do mean? I didn't go to the drive-in yesterday."

He said it with such an innocent look that had I not been with Winston and Anita and actually seen them with my own eyes, I would have believed him.

"I KNOW you went and you had someone with you, Dougie. Who was it?"

"No, whoever told you I was with another girl is lying—it's not true!"

It was hard to accept the fact that he was outright lying to me. It cut deep because he was the only person I could depend on during such uncertain times. My heart started racing, but outwardly I was calm.

"Someone didn't tell me. I SAW you when Winston took Anita and I out for a drive yesterday."

Dougie stared at me with the look of a child who had been caught with its hand in the cookie jar. For a brief moment I almost felt sorry for him. He seemed desperate to find some excuse, so I sort of let him off the hook by changing the subject.

"Do you think we can go over to Lingan Road so I can drive the car before I go home?" I asked.

"Oh, okay!"

He seemed relieved at my suggestion. I managed to hide my feelings of hurt and disappointment for the next half hour or so that we spent together. But I had a sleepless night agonizing over whether or not I should even continue going out with him. I was torn.

We never did see or hear from Justine, George or Mama while we were living on Plummer Avenue with that family, and I often wondered why. Then one day as Anita and I were talking to our best friend Mary in front of Eaton's, we happened to see Justine and George drive by. But as they passed in front of us either they didn't see us or they pretended not to, so I was puzzled and felt hurt when we didn't hear from them anymore.

A few months later when school ended, Anita and I moved from that family's place on Plummer Avenue to be with Mama, who had been staying with her sister Christie Ling. She was a retired nurse who lived in a lovely large yellow house on Ling Street just behind our school. Her husband had passed away a few years ago and her adult daughter was living with her. Mama had moved in with them at the same time Anita and I went to board with the family our parish priest had found for us.

Anyway, we heard that Justine and George had finally been able to adopt a baby as they had planned to do a while back. We were thrilled to receive the news that they'd soon welcome the newborn baby home with them. Christie and her daughter were so kind while Anita, Mama and I stayed there for a couple of months.

By the end of that summer, Anita and I found out we would be moving away from New Waterford, but no one knew where. Meantime, Dougie and I continued to see each other on a regular basis as I chose to believe that he was going out with me and no one else.

Something just popped into my mind regarding an incident that took place while we were living there on Ling Street. It happened just before we moved away from New Waterford. Anita couldn't find her sandals when we were getting ready to go to church one Sunday morning, and we were rushing so we wouldn't be late. So when Anita couldn't find them, Mama handed her a pair of her chunky-heeled shoes and said, "Here, put these on."

"NO! They're too big for me!" Anita protested.

Mama became flustered, took both shoes and placed them at Anita's feet, saying, "Here, you have to wear these. We don't have anything else."

She made her put them on and quickly ushered us out the door. Anita protested all the way across the schoolyard and to the church, but to no avail. While squabbling over the shoes, they didn't notice a couple of girls whom I recognized as being Grade 10 high school students. They giggled when Anita tried to walk properly.

"Walk faster, we're going to be late!" Mama insisted.

I felt so sorry for Anita. When she realized that the older girls were watching, she stopped and in a burst of anger, said, "NO! I'M NOT GOING!"

"Yes, you are," Mama said in a calm, determined voice.

She then grabbed Anita's arm and slapped her across the face.

Needless to say, the students were shocked to see such a display of insensitivity on Mama's part. In tears, poor Anita kicked the shoes off to the side and ran across the schoolyard and back towards Ling Street. I just wanted to disappear.

"Come on, we're late," Mama said. "Mass must have started by now!"

The girls walked around us as they passed, glancing back with a look of disbelief. I followed Mama inside the church as she strutted down the aisle in her typical calm attitude as if nothing had happened.

As usual, the next day nothing was mentioned about the incident. We simply went about our day as if everything was normal. This had been the pattern over the years—everything was simply swept under the rug. None of us were able to either question or complain when treated badly.

Anita and I didn't hear anything about when we were to move away until about two days before the actual event. Even though we were expecting to leave New Waterford sometime that fall, the news still seemed rather sudden to me once I was told. I must have called Dougie the moment I heard about it because the next thing I remember was Dougie and I sitting in his car near the cliff overlooking the ocean at the end of our street. I was touched by his emotional state, which showed he must have had deep feelings for me. He was near tears when I told him. No one had ever had feelings for me like this before, and even though I can't recall shedding any tears, I do remember feeling a deep sadness when we parted. I knew I would miss him terribly, but I felt helpless to do anything.

Chapter 7

The next day, Mama, Anita and I were driven to the Sydney airport where we were to have our very first flight on an airplane. We were seventeen years old by then, but we looked and acted more like we were around fourteen. We never did mature at par with other teenagers. It's rather strange, but I can't remember the trip itself; there was no excitement or expectation that I can recall.

Our older brother Jimmy, who seemed more like a stranger to us, picked us up in Montreal. There was no sign of affection whatsoever, and only a few words were spoken between Jimmy and Mama as we drove to our destination. We were staying at Tony's place, a duplex not far from downtown Montreal. Tony, who was just two years older than Anita and me, apparently had an agreement with Mama that we were to stay with him and his girlfriend Rosemary, whom he later married and had children with. They were open to having us there, but, from the few bits of conversation I heard, we were to find work as soon as possible.

I believe Mama stayed only a couple of days in Montreal before she went on to Toronto to live with our sister Yvonne, the one who liked singing and cleaning the house when she lived at home in New Waterford. She left for Toronto at an early age, as most members of our family did, and was married to an easy-going guy from Nova Scotia. They had two little girls. Yvonne now enjoyed singing in a western nightclub in Toronto, and both she and her husband worked as superintendents in a high-rise apartment building in a nice suburban area of Toronto.

Mama was to live with them permanently and have her own room, which was tastefully done by Yvonne (who liked quality as Mama did). The living room had all French provincial style furniture with a marble coffee table, etc., and her place was kept clean and inviting. This was very appealing to Mama, and I could see she was really looking forward to living there.

Mama asked Jimmy if he would take her to see St. Joseph's Oratory, a Catholic basilica and national shrine on Mount Royal, before she left. It didn't matter much to me, but the four of us went. That's all I remember, really; it was a non-event in my mind. Anita told me only recently over the phone what happened. She said we were standing in the kitchen of Tony's apartment when apparently I made some kind of a remark that Jimmy did not like, so he just reached out and slapped me hard in the face. When I started to cry, Anita said she looked at Mama and said, "He just hit Anna!"

"They're too sensitive," Jimmy said. "Look at them cross-eyed and they cry."

According to Anita, Mama just stood there pretending not to see what just took place right there in front of her. She didn't say a word. I wasn't all that surprised that Jimmy would do such a thing, but I was shocked that I couldn't remember it.

When Mama left us there with Tony and Rosemary, Anita and I didn't have a clue as to how to navigate our way around Montreal let alone where to start looking for work.

A couple of days after we arrived, Anita had taken out her art lessons she had begun just before leaving New Waterford. The moment Tony came in from work, he said, "Get that junk off the table, we have to get supper." Of course, Anita immediately complied. Being spoken to in this manner was nothing new.

It didn't take long for Rosemary to see that we really did not know how to get started with our new life there in Montreal. That we needed some help. So she called a relative who had just left a job as an elevator operator at the Queen Elizabeth, a new high-class hotel in downtown Montreal. After a short conversation with her about us, she turned to us and said, "Go to the personnel department right away to apply for that position before somebody else does—you just might get the job."

The next morning, Anita and I took the bus for the very first time and found our way to the hotel. We did not expect things to move so quickly. We were shown around the hotel and to where the lockers were, where to punch our cards when coming in and leaving the hotel, measured for our uniforms, and even given a medical exam. We were told to show up the next morning half an hour before starting work at eight o'clock.

Anita told me that when she was examined by the hotel doctor, he said her pelvis was tipped and that if she ever had children, they would have to be delivered by cesarian section. I immediately thought about that time when she was injured while playing in the Miller's yard when I had to help her get home. Could that have been the cause?

As elevator operators, it was pointed out that we would have to do shift work which changed every two weeks in rotation. We did the day shift from 8 a.m. to 4 p.m., and night shift from 4 p.m. to midnight. Tony and Rosemary were clearly happy when we got back with the news that we both had been hired that day.

After just over two weeks since arriving in Montreal, Anita and I not only had work, but we found a small but nice furnished apartment just a few minutes away by bus from the Queen Elizabeth Hotel. We soon realized that it was too expensive, so we looked for another place we could afford. Fortunately, we were able to rent another apartment not that far away. We were more than happy to take it and got settled in without much hassle.

An incident shortly afterwards made us think twice about living there. We had just finished our 4 p.m. to midnight shift, and as we got off the bus and started walking down the short dead-end street to where our apartment was, I noticed a shadow of someone coming up right behind us. It moved so quietly and swiftly that I didn't have a chance to turn around before my purse was suddenly snatched away from me! Panic-stricken, we ran towards our apartment building as he disappeared into the alleyway with it. Reaching the entrance, breathless and on the verge of tears, Anita nervously fumbled with her keys. It hit me then that he not only had my wallet but my keys as well!

"Good thing I have mine!" she said, "otherwise we'd be locked out!"

When she said this, I flashed back to when we were locked out at home and ended up walking to Adeline's place and sleeping on their back step. The moment we stepped into our apartment, we drew the curtains, pushed the couch in front of the door and made sure it was securely locked before going to bed.

The next day as we left for work, I spotted something on the ground halfway down the alleyway.

"Do you think that could be my purse?" I said as I gingerly walked over to check.

Sure enough, there it was. My wallet was missing, as I expected, but I was surprised to find my keys were still inside. This lifted my spirit slightly, but we really did not want to stay there anymore. From then on, whenever we'd get off the bus and start walking to our apartment, we'd find ourselves constantly checking behind to make sure nobody was following us.

I found it intimidating to be in the cafeteria with some of the other employees at the Queen Elizabeth Hotel. Aside from the fact that we had Cape Breton accents, we were twins when dressed in our uniforms and sometimes it felt as if we were some kind of a target. This particular bellboy, who was actually a married man with children, seemed to take pleasure in teasing us whenever we happened to be in the cafeteria. He always smiled when he came over, pulled up a chair and began the conversation with rude comments about our accents. So it wasn't very long before I started to go downstairs to Central Station (the train station) on my break to have my burger or whatever just to avoid seeing him.

Dougie sent me a small black portable radio and a pair of fur-lined leather gloves for Christmas. During one of my twenty-minute breaks, I was lying down on a long wooden bench between two rows of lockers listening to music on my radio when I suddenly realized I only had two minutes left before I had to be back at work. In my rush to stuff the radio and gloves into the locker, I didn't see that it didn't lock properly when I closed it. So when I returned at the end of my shift, both the radio and gloves were missing. I was disappointed but not upset about it; I figured out what must have happened and just accepted it.

Once in a while, Dougie and I wrote a short note just to let each other know what was happening. In one of them he told me he was planning to come to Montreal for a visit in the summertime. I was so happy to hear that, and it helped keep me going through the rest of that winter.

Because of the shift work, I was extremely tired at times. I was in awe at some of the other elevator operators who would finish their four to midnight shifts and still be able to go out to nightclubs afterwards—even when they had to get up for a morning shift the next day. All Anita and I could think about was getting to bed to have enough energy to get back to the elevators the next day. I developed dark circles under my eyes after only six months on the job.

Even if we did have the energy after finishing a night shift, we had no desire to go out afterwards. Actually one of the operators remarked that we were odd or strange because of this.

Teenage idol Fabian stayed overnight in the hotel one time. Anita and I happened to be working the night shift, and she told me that as he came into her elevator with his crew, he smiled at her and asked, "What is your name?" She said she was surprised when he leaned over and whispered his room number in her ear. The next day when the other elevator operators heard about this, they actually did not believe her, especially when she said that she wasn't interested in going up to his room after her shift was finished at midnight. Anita said they thought she must be crazy to have declined because, after all, this was "FABIAN"!

We didn't go anywhere; life was just working on the elevators and that was it. We both felt terribly lonely in the city because we never heard a word from Mama or the rest of the family. We felt abandoned. However, we knew we had to accept the reality that this was our life now and we might as well get used to it.

When the snow finally melted and spring was well on its way, I got a phone call out of the blue from Dougie. I was so happy to hear his voice and equally as surprised when he told me he had just arrived in Montreal and was staying with a couple of his friends from New Waterford. When he came to our apartment, I was really excited to see him again, but later my brother Jimmy showed up! The one who slapped me in the face! *What in the world is he doing here?* I thought. *And how did he know where we live?* But with Dougie being there, I quickly let go of any concerns and tried to be polite at least.

As I chatted with Dougie about his plans, I wondered if he would be staying in Montreal to find work or if he was just visiting. Anita reminded me that we had to leave for the night shift soon, but I decided to stay home because Dougie had just come all the way from Cape Breton to be with me. He brought his friend's sleeping bag with him because I told him that we only had a bachelor apartment. At least it was furnished and had a couch that turned into a bed.

Once the initial excitement of our meeting wore off, I became very uncomfortable with Jimmy being there. It was getting late, so I asked him if he would please leave. He just ignored me as if I wasn't even there and kept asking Dougie's questions about his work in the mines. This went on for quite some time. Dougie didn't seem to know what to say when he saw I was beginning to get annoyed. I could tell he wasn't sure whether I was upset with him or with Jimmy. But it was obvious that I was tired and just wanted to call it a night.

I said I was going to have my shower and told Jimmy again that I wanted him gone by the time I was finished. I took twice as long as usual, but when I came out of the bathroom he was still there—he hadn't budged. So in sheer frustration I pulled the couch down into a bed, threw my blankets on top and rolled up into a ball. Before I knew it, I was out like a light.

I don't know what time it was, but during the night I woke up from sheer shock when I found Jimmy spooning me on the couch. He was rubbing his fingers on my vagina and whispering, "Shush, be quiet!" He tried to hold me down, but I jumped up, grabbed my pillow and ran for the bathroom, locking the door behind me. I was shaking all over. I caught a glimpse of Dougie as I almost tripped over him while trying to get away. He was rolled up in his sleeping bag on the floor snoring loudly. I felt like I was losing my mind. I didn't know what to do next.

I put the towels into the bathtub along with my pillow and stayed there until Anita got back from work. She knocked on the bathroom door and asked in a hushed tone, "How long are you going to be in there?" I opened it slowly while checking to make sure Jimmy was gone. Thankfully, he was by then. Dougie was still asleep on the floor. When Anita went into the bathroom, I couldn't wait to get back to bed and was sound asleep within minutes.

Believe it or not, I didn't tell Dougie or Anita about my horrible experience that night. Maybe out of shame or embarrassment, I don't know, but to this day I still get angry at the thought of what happened. In the morning, I did my best to act as if nothing happened and forced myself to take part in small talk between Anita and Dougie, which was mainly about him and his friends from back home.

Dougie told me about a week later that he was looking for work in Montreal, and I jumped for joy to know he would actually do this. I had no expectations when he came to visit me, but I secretly hoped it could happen. He said one of his friends from back home made more money working in Montreal than he did working in the mines. So Dougie decided to go with him and apply for a job working on Montreal's Jacques Cartier Bridge. The men were lowered inside a huge square cement box into the Saint-Lawrence River where they had to repair pillars that supported the bridge. I was told miners were always accepted because of their experience working underground, but I was concerned for Dougie's safety. Not that working in the pit wasn't dangerous, of course it was, but to hear that they could suddenly experience bleeding from the ears, eyes or nose while under compressed air working there under the river made me very uneasy.

It wasn't long before Dougie was earning a good salary at the Jacques Cartier Bridge and things seemed to be working out for the both of us. However, it was getting more difficult for me to cope with the rotating shifts on the elevators. The physical exhaustion was too much to handle at times, and it was the same for Anita.

I finished my eight to four shift one day and decided to drop in to see Dougie and his friends from New Waterford. I had never gone there before. They were happy to see me, but I really wasn't in a chatty mood. Actually I was feeling down and just needed to be with Dougie for a while. Dougie, his friend Martin and his girlfriend Annie were in good humour, so I faked a smile and sat down at the table with them. I was pretty tired, so when I was unable to keep up my charade any longer, I asked if they wouldn't mind if I were to go into the living room and lay down on their couch.

"Sure, go ahead," said Martin.

They were talking and the loud laughter was starting to get to me. I was feeling lonely and needed Dougie to come and sit by my side, so I went into the kitchen and asked if he would come into the living room with me, which he did. But after a couple of minutes he suggested I have a snooze, and he went back to join the others. I started to think maybe I should leave since Dougie seemed to prefer to have their company over mine. Either that or else he just didn't pick up on my emotional need at the time. After maybe fifteen minutes or so, I got up and went into the kitchen.

"Are you okay?" asked Dougie.

"Oh yes, I'll be fine," I lied, and I joined in on the laughter.

A couple of minutes later, as I was standing next to Dougie who was sitting at the table, I realized I was unable to stop laughing. I was slowly doubling over while leaning against the fridge as if I were about to fall down. My laughter turned into tears, and I began sobbing uncontrollably. Dougie reached out to grab me before I hit the floor, but I screamed and pushed him away.

Next thing I remember was I inside an ambulance. I had no idea what was happening to me.

I don't remember getting the needle that put me asleep, but after spending one night in the Montreal General Hospital, I was told I could leave. I took a couple of days off work trying to get my strength back so I could return, but I was afraid I would lose my job if I didn't get back soon.

Meantime, I sat down and wrote a note to Mama telling her what had happened. I honestly did not expect a response from her, but I just wanted to let her know what was happening, I guess. I don't remember her contacting us, but she did come over to Montreal shortly after that and stayed for a few days. We had already moved into another apartment by then, which had a bedroom, was furnished and quite nice with the new drapes that Anita and I bought.

Mama seemed to approve, however, when we left for work it didn't feel right that she was there all by herself. And I remember how uncomfortable it was when Dougie came by to see me because they disliked each other. He used to refer to her as the blue-haired witch. Just before she returned to Toronto, when Dougie happened to be saying good night at the door, she said under her breath, "You should go back to the woods where you belong." I was glad when she left because I couldn't get rid of the memories of when we were in New Waterford and how she never wanted to be around us.

In August, almost a year after we arrived in Montreal, I noticed how much Dougie missed his family back in Cape Breton. It was the haying season, the time of year when Dougie used to work out in the fields with his family. Even though he had his buddies with him there in Montreal and was making a really good salary, I sensed it was only a matter of time before he would go back to Cape Breton. I was right, but I wasn't prepared emotionally for how to handle it when it actually did happen. I had anticipated that we would talk about it and that he would kind of reassure me that we would stay connected at all times. But he didn't say a word about it, not even on the day before he planned to leave.

I couldn't believe the casual way in which he brought it up one Saturday after having lunch together. We were sitting outside on my balcony. He gave me no hint at all that he had decided to leave Montreal—like, that very day! I had no idea until the very last minute. As we got to the door, he hugged me for an unusually long time and with much more emotion than usual. Then, with a serious look on his face he said, "I have to get going because Martin is supposed to meet me at one o'clock. We're heading back home and I don't want to get caught in the rush hour traffic."

"WHAT? But? But?" I stuttered. I couldn't believe my ears. "You mean you're really leaving Montreal today? Like right NOW?"

"Yes, I picked up my pay cheque yesterday and told them I wouldn't be going back on Monday."

I felt a wave of sadness wash over me. I didn't know what to say or what to do. It was so matter of fact—and so sudden! I think I went into a sort of panic mode for a second, and I found myself saying, "But I don't want to stay here without you! If you're going, I want to go too!"

He didn't seem to know what to say.

"But where would you stay if you came back with us?"

"Maybe Justine would let me stay at her place for a while," I said.

"Well, you could call her and find out."

But then I thought, *What if she says no?*

"I think I'll let her know I'm coming when we're already on our way," I said.

Dougie hesitated for a moment and said, "All right. But I don't know if that's such a good idea."

Before he had a chance to persuade me to change my mind, I grabbed a pen and scribbled a note to Anita, who was out shopping for groceries. I quickly threw some clothes into an overnight bag and said, "I'm ready!"

I left my apartment keys along with the note on the kitchen cupboard as we left. It did not feel right to leave Anita in such a predicament, but my mind was spinning at top speed and the only thing I could think of was being with Dougie. When Anita found the note, she didn't know what to do. She called Yvonne in Toronto who told her to come there, that she should not stay in Montreal by herself.

So Anita and I were living apart for the first time in our lives. Thankfully, Justine allowed me to stay at her place. Dougie went back to work in the pit right after finishing with the haying season.

Once in a while, Anita and I sent a short note just to keep in touch. She mentioned that there was a guy named Chris from Denmark who had asked her out. He was a good friend of the family, but he was fifteen years older than her. And that was it; she didn't fill me in on any of the details, so I just assumed she must be going out with him.

A couple of months passed before we connected again, and I assumed she was going out with him. I wrote to tell her that I did not get my period in October and that it was possible I was pregnant. Instead of the short note I'd usually get, I received an frantic three-page letter describing her current situation. Her opening line was: "ME TOO! I missed my October period!" My eyes popped wide open and I felt my chin drop. *Oh my GOD! We are both pregnant at the same time!* The only difference was that I had not told anyone except Dougie. Anita had already let Yvonne know, who then, of course, told Mama.

Chapter 8

Anita said that when Mama saw her the next day she was upset with her.

"Anna wouldn't get into trouble like that!" she said.

To which Anita responded, "Anna is too!"

Anita said Mama was extremely disappointed in both of us. She actually liked Chris and thought he would be good for Anita so, even though she was disappointed, Mama encouraged Anita to go ahead and marry Chris. I can understand her thinking at that time: Chris was older and had a steady job; he would be able to take care of her, plus he was a friend of the family.

She said Yvonne offered to take care of everything should they go ahead and get married. After a few letters back and forth, Yvonne told her that she would arrange everything for me, too, if I wanted to have a double ring ceremony there in Toronto. After talking it over with Dougie, he thought it would be a good idea then for us to go to Toronto. But his family didn't think so, and it became apparent when none of them showed up for the wedding. I was more concerned about the timing since Anita and I would be showing soon and we still had to find dresses.

Everything was a blur. I vaguely remember Yvonne taking us to a shop that rented bridal gowns and finding two that fit properly. The double ring ceremony was memorable though. As Chris was about to put the ring on Anita's finger, she suddenly fainted. She just sank to the floor. She was helped up and asked if she was okay to continue. She nodded, but I was concerned. Did she really want to get married that day? Maybe she wasn't sure but felt it was the proper thing to do because she was pregnant? I couldn't help but wonder.

I knew I wanted to marry Dougie and have our baby. But at the same time, I would have preferred to avoid the wedding part because I was so terribly shy and insecure. None the less I was truly grateful that Yvonne took this on, organizing everything as she did.

When we all went from the church to Yvonne's apartment for the reception, there was Yvonne's husband Tom, their two little girls, Jenny Anne and Ada, Mama, and a few friends of the family. It was a nice small gathering where everyone seemed genuinely happy for us.

While in the kitchen preparing some drinks for everyone, Yvonne handed me a drink that smelled like alcohol.

"Here, this will help you relax."

I think it had some orange juice mixed in. I took it to be polite, but my stomach had a slight burning sensation immediately. Mama passed through the kitchen at that moment and sort of frowned at Yvonne but said nothing, then she turned to me and said, "Never say no to your husband," and walked away. I thought it was kind of funny, as if we were back in the days when women were conditioned to be passive. Or maybe she was just repeating her own mother's advice given on the day she married Papa? Anyway, everyone seemed to be supportive. Even Yvonne's friend who was out of town offered their apartment for Dougie and I to stay in that night. We were anxious to get on the road back to Cape Breton because there was a snowstorm in the forecast for Toronto the very next day, so we left right away.

When we finally arrived in New Waterford after our long drive from Toronto, we stayed with Justine and George in my childhood home on Mahon Street. Since there were four bedrooms and only two were being used, they said we could stay there until we found a place to live. The baby they had adopted, a cute blond, blue-eyed little boy named Patrick, was almost a year old, and I was happy we were able to share some time with them.

On weekends, Justine and George often played cards at the kitchen table, and they invited us to play along one Saturday. Dougie declined saying he had already promised to give his brother a hand. He lived out on Roaches Road with his mother, which was where Dougie lived before going to Montreal. I had no problem with that, and I stayed and joined in on the game. Just before going downstairs to play cards, I looked at my shape sideways in the mirror and thought I'd try on my new black maternity skirt and matching top. Even though I was just beginning to show slightly, I was picturing being full term and ready to give birth. I opened the drawer and took out the baby clothes that Justine had bought for me and held up the tiny little T-shirts, marvelling at the size. *I can't believe I will have a baby soon and will dress him or her in these tiny little shirts*, I mused.

Justine commented on how she liked my new outfit when I sat down to start playing Scat with them. Not long into the game, I felt some slight pressure in my abdomen but ignored it as I was concentrating on my next move. George noticed I was beginning to squirm slightly and asked if it might be more comfortable for me to sit on a cushion. I thanked him and got right back into the game—I was about to win this round! Totally focused, I picked the card I needed to win and held up my hand saying, "Scat!" "Then ouch! a sudden pinch of pain caused me to bend over". I put the cards down, clutched my belly and gently laid my head on the table.

"What's wrong?" Justine asked. "Do you have some pain"?

A second later it was gone, so I didn't want to move in case it came back. As I regained my composure and sat upright again, I could see they were afraid for me, so I jokingly reassured them with, "Don't worry, I'm not going into labour now. It's much too early for that; I'm only four months along. Want to play another hand?" I asked cheerfully.

"Well, if you'd like maybe we'll play one more round," said George. "What do you think, Justine?"

She looked a bit concerned when I took the deck in my hands and started shuffling the cards.

Ten minutes later, I had another pinch of pain exactly like the first one.

"Ouch!" I said, "Oh, oh, maybe I'd better stop now."

"Yes, maybe you should lie down on the couch," said Justine as she helped me up out of the chair.

The pain left but I felt a tightness in my abdomen and started to worry. George and Justine were now debating whether or not I should go to the hospital when I heard George on the phone saying, "Okay, we'll be there in a few minutes."

Everything seemed to move quickly when we got to the hospital. There was a silver metal stand next to my bed that had a plastic pouch hanging from it and a tube running down to my arm with a needle stuck in my hand. The nurse made me feel comfortable and cared for, and somehow I knew everything was going to be all right. The doctor came in later and told me I had experienced a "threatened miscarriage." He said that because we were only minutes away from the hospital and had called them right away, they were able to prevent it. I was so thankful that Justine and George were there for me that day, and I was relieved when Dougie came to take me back to their place that evening.

I still had almost five months left, so we started to look for a place of our own. My friend Mary, who lived next to Eaton's department store, told us about an apartment that had recently become vacant in the same building, so we went and checked it out. We ended up taking it because it was not expensive, and I liked the idea of living close to Mary and her family again.

I had my first contraction on June 29. At my previous doctor's appointment I was told the baby could come either before or after that date. And that sometimes a mother could experience what is called a false labour, where she might have a few contractions but then they could suddenly stop. What I understood was that it wasn't always necessary to go to the hospital right away, but from the first contraction I just knew it was the real thing. I started to get ready.

It was just after breakfast, and I was alone because Dougie had left for his mother's place on Roaches Road where he was supposed to change a tire on his car. When I called there, his mother said he left for Sydney with his brother right after they changed the tire. She would let him know the minute he got back. There were no cell phones or texting in those days, so when the labour pains started, I called Justine. She said George would pick me up if I wanted to go over to her place while in labour.

"Yes, I don't want to be alone here," I said.

I took my packed suitcase and waited for George. I was so grateful I didn't have to be alone! Justine had never given birth either, so we were both excited that my contractions had actually started. At the same time, I was a little nervous when the contractions became more intense and frequent.

"Why isn't Dougie calling me?"

I tried to ignore my fears by repeating to myself: *Whatever is meant to happen will happen! Worrying about it will not change the outcome.* That mindset helped keep me calm, but it seemed like an eternity before Dougie got back and we finally headed for the hospital.

As we came into the lobby, Dougie was walking ahead of me too quickly and paying no attention to me whatsoever. When the elevator doors opened, a nurse was there with a wheelchair, greeting us with a smile as if she had been expecting us. To my surprise and disappointment, Dougie just handed my suitcase to her, turned to me and said, "Okay hon, I'll see you later." He waved to me as the elevator doors closed. I tried not to show it, but I was obviously embarrassed at the way he abruptly left me there. The nurse quickly stepped in with reassuring words of encouragement as she wheeled me towards my room.

After twelve hours in labour and the nurse gently coaching me on that last push, all I can remember was being awfully tired and praying the pain would stop. That's when I heard, "It's a boy!" I expected to hear a robust first cry but nothing happened. I held my breath … waiting. After a moment or two came his little voice that sounded more like a whimper. They quickly wrapped him in a blanket but didn't place him in my arms as you'd see happen in the movies. The nurse held him up, but I could only see his tiny face, which had a sort of reddish tinge and a head full of black hair. His eyes were half closed and squinting. He looked so cute, yawning as if ready to fall asleep in the cocoon-like blanket he was wrapped in.

When they started wheeling me out of the delivery room, I heard someone ask how I was doing. I was a bit groggy and didn't see anyone as they moved me along the hallway. But I did recognize the voice as being that of Dougie's sister Olga. I remember mumbling in a low tone, "Never again. Never again!"

"Oh they all say that!" she laughed … then they're back again the next year!"

I was in no mood for jokes.

"Where's Dougie? Why isn't he here?" I asked.

I fell asleep as soon as they took me to my room. Later, I woke up to the sound of the nurse talking to someone who was sitting next to my bed. I turned to see it was Dougie. He said he had been to see the baby already and wanted to know if I was okay. But he didn't stay long. We had decided while I was pregnant that if it was a boy, we would give him Papa's name, Andrew. His family started to call him Andy from day one, which was just fine with me.

We had rented that apartment next to Mary's place for the summer, but by the fall Dougie decided we should move to Roaches Road on the outskirts of town where his family lived. It was mid-October 1962. I was twenty years old and Dougie was twenty one.

On the left side of the driveway was the house where Dougie used to live with his mother and older brother Ewen, the one who rode a sulky in the harness races in Sydney. Just behind that was the barn where their three racehorses were kept. On the right side of the driveway was the little bungalow where Dougie's other brother Hartigan lived with his wife Georgie and their two children. They had recently added another little room on the back that you couldn't see from the driveway.

It was decided that we would live there temporarily if we finished it off on the inside. I thought, *Okay, I'll make the best of the situation at hand and will do whatever I can to help.* Andy wasn't walking yet, and Hartigan's wife Georgie and I did get along reasonably well. She said she'd keep an eye on Andy for me by leaving her kitchen door open when I would be busy working in the room.

When Dougie and Hartigan had finished stuffing the pink insulation in between the studs and nailing large pieces of cardboard over it, I had this idea to paste wallpaper over it all. So I got right to it and was totally wrapped up in trying to finish the job before the cold weather arrived. Before I knew it, Christmas Eve was upon us and there I was, knee-deep in wallpapering with Andy under foot needing my attention at the same time.

I don't know where Dougie was, but I will never forget how embarrassed I was when, without any warning, Mary, whom I hadn't seen since we moved out of the apartment next to her place, dropped by. I was standing on a little stepladder after pulling the last sheet of wallpaper up out of the water, ready to paste it onto the wall. My arms were stretched upwards holding it by the edges while straining to get it straight along the top when I heard a gentle knock on the door.

"Come in!" I said, rather impatiently.

I heard the door open and close. Unable to move or else I'd lose my balance, I managed a "Hi!" while pressing the wallpaper in place. But there was no response. As I turned to see who had come in, I almost fell over.

"MARY!" I exclaimed, gripping the ladder to steady myself as I carefully stepped down.

Both of us were speechless. My mind snapped a picture of her in that moment. Instead of her usual plain Jane look, she looked rather striking in a lovely black cloth coat with a bright red corsage on the lapel. Her natural light blond hair stood out against her black coat. In her typical calm, demure manner, she stood there for a second or two scanning the room with a look of empathy in her big soft blue eyes.

"Maybe I should have called before coming?" she said with an apologetic tone.

She was obviously embarrassed to have stepped into such a mess, but not as much as I was. How tired and haggard I must have looked, especially with this being Christmas Eve and all. She reached into her purse and pulled out a small square package with a little ribbon on top.

"Merry Christmas," she said, handing it to me with a warm smile.

Then she turned to Andy and gave him a little toy, which kept him busy for the next while. I gave her a big hug in appreciation for having thought of me on that Christmas Eve. She didn't stay long, maybe ten minutes at the most.

Her short visit gave me the boost of energy I needed to finish the job before going to bed that night. I fell into bed exhausted but at the same time satisfied that I had finished the job. I was glad Mary had stopped by despite the embarrassing situation she walked into. I opened the gift the next morning. It was a cute little bracelet she had made herself. I smiled, promising myself I would find the time to visit with her and her family more often.

As time went on, things were not working out as we had hoped on Roaches Road. Not only did I become pregnant again when Andy was only four months old, but the place was not heated properly. I had to keep checking on Andy during the night to make sure the mitts I put on his little hands didn't come off. I bundled him up with lots of blankets and prayed he wouldn't catch a cold. I was not happy there at all, and by the end of

January when Andy was just over six months old, he caught pneumonia and had to stay in the hospital for two whole weeks.

As things went from bad to worse, I felt a division opening between Dougie's family and me. And when I discovered I was pregnant again, I didn't even mention it to them. I don't recall having any discussion with Dougie regarding what we were going to do or where we would go from there either. I realized I had created a more problematic situation by becoming pregnant again, and I turned on myself, wondering *What is wrong with me!* There was no use talking to Dougie about how I felt because he was not open to listening. Besides, I found he confided in his family whenever he had something on his mind, which always left me feeling like an outsider.

By the time spring arrived, it was obvious to everyone that I was expecting again. Dougie must have talked to his family about what we should do because out of the blue both he and Olga wanted me to go with them to look at a small bungalow for sale in Scotchtown, which was on the outskirts of New Waterford. I was so excited at the thought that we might buy our own little house, and I couldn't wait to see it for myself.

When we pulled into the driveway, it looked like an average small bungalow on a small lot. There were houses on both sides that were similar in appearance and size. As we got out of the car, I was thinking how wonderful it would be if we were to buy this little house! Walking towards the back step, I could see it needed a paint job, *But that shouldn't be a problem*, I thought as I started my assessment. We entered through the back porch and came into the kitchen. Even though the rooms were very small, it was much better than Roaches Road. With two bedrooms the kids could have their own room. Then it hit me …

"Where's the bathroom?" I asked.

Dougie and Olga glanced at each other.

"We have to have a bathroom. Why would we buy a house without one?"

I was beginning to have mixed feelings about this whole idea.

"It has an outhouse we can use until we put the bathroom in," Dougie said. "I'll start to dig a trench from the house to the street right away so I can put the sewer pipe in."

I wanted to believe him, but based on what he would say and what he would actually do, I was afraid to go along with it.

"Couldn't we look for another place instead?" I pleaded like a child.

"No, this one's a bargain," he insisted. "It's not possible to find another house for the price I paid for this one."

"What? You mean you bought it already?"

I wasn't sure how to react about their choice and the fact that I had no say in the matter. This annoyed me to no end.

Chapter 9

Dougie's intention to dig the trench may have been good when we first moved in, but then he quickly lost interest and I started to worry, since I was not able to do anything about it. I refused to use the outhouse, I absolutely hated it. I'd take a pail half full of water and use that. Then I'd place a thick square piece of plywood over the top and leave it in the porch. When it was dark outside, I'd take it to the outhouse because I felt so ashamed. It is difficult enough to sit on a toilet properly when almost full term, but squatting over a pail?

When I put Andy outside to play, attaching him to the back step with a rope so he couldn't wander off, I saw my neighbour for the first time. She was out in her backyard working in a vegetable garden and looked to be around my age. I wanted to meet her but felt a little shy, so I went into the house to find something to give to her to break the ice.

I came back with a set of pillowslips that had never been opened and walked over.

"Hi, my name is Anna," I said.

She looked up at me with a serious *What do you want?* expression on her face that set me back a little.

"I have these pillowslips I thought you might like to have," I said as I stretched out my arm to give them to her over the fence.

She got up slowly and came over as if I was bothering her. She told me her name as she took the package and turned away. I stood there for a moment feeling embarrassed for trying to make the connection with her. I went back into the house.

I never did see her after that, but I did meet my other neighbour not long after that. I was eight months pregnant and happened to be down on my knees scrubbing the floor in the kitchen surrounded by the strong aroma of the industrial Pine-Sol I was using.

"Oh no, you shouldn't be doing that!" she said with concern in her voice.

I struggled to stand upright, turning to see a short middle-aged woman with little sparkling blue eyes smiling at me. She was standing in the doorway.

"Baby is coming soon and look at you!"

After introducing herself, we had a friendly chat. To my surprise, she invited me over to her place when I finished to have a shower. As soon as I finished the floor, I happily got my towel, grabbed Andy and went over. Her husband, a short, muscular man with an accent, was also friendly. They were both from Czechoslovakia. They clearly loved children and made a big fuss over Andy, which made me feel very welcome in their little home. I was truly grateful for their kindness and their insisting that I come back to use their shower.

"Don't be shy!" they said with a smile as I left.

I was beginning to feel terribly anxious as my time grew closer. On June 29, Andy turned one year old, which meant I would be going into the hospital to give birth again. Not having a bathroom in the house was something I knew I'd have to face when I brought the baby home.

I also had to use the scrubbing board, as they called it, to wash our clothes by hand when we first moved into the house. It had a wooden frame around thick, wavy glass, and I had to take each piece of clothing, rub the bar of soap on it and start scrubbing. I did this for about two weeks before Dougie bought a second-hand wringer washer to use.

The energy needed to deal with everything wore me down, so my challenge was figuring out how to cope once I brought our newborn home in just a couple of weeks' time.

On July 18, 1963, I gave birth to a baby girl whom we named Elizabeth Anne, after Dougie's mother. Even though I was concerned about how I'd manage with a one-year-old and an infant when I got home, I was thankful they were both healthy. I was determined to do my best to take good care of them.

I shared a semi-private room with another young mother, and we were having a conversation regarding our deliveries; they turned out to be only hours apart the day before. Our conversation was interrupted when we heard a commotion in the hallway outside our room. A nurse came running past the door pulling what looked like a grey tank on wheels.

"Someone must be having a problem," I said.

We walked towards the door to get a peek, but everyone had disappeared, so we got back into our beds and continued on with our conversation.

I don't know how long it was after that, maybe 10 minutes or so, when a nurse walked into our room looking rather serious and pulled the drape dividing our beds. She said my baby was having some trouble breathing and was turning blue so they had to give her some oxygen.

"But don't worry," the nurse said. "We took care of it and she is sleeping comfortably now. We will bring her to you in a few minutes, okay?"

"You mean that was *my* baby that needed that oxygen tank we saw the nurse running with?" I asked.

"Yes, but she will be just fine."

I thanked her for reassuring me, but I wondered why we didn't inquire to find out if either one of our babies might have been in danger. I guess we automatically assumed it was someone else having a problem, not us. I was uneasy and thinking maybe I wasn't a good mother, but then I forgave myself and promised I'd be more attentive once I had her home with me.

I was glad Dougie's family took good care of Andy while I was in the hospital. They even kept him for a couple of days after I brought Elizabeth Anne home, which was a big help. I guess they couldn't help but see the huge challenge ahead, and they knew Dougie didn't finish digging the trench as he had promised. I was told Andy had taken his first steps while I was in the hospital. He was not out of diapers yet, and with Elizabeth Anne just starting, I knew I had to brace myself for what laid ahead.

Early each morning after taking care of the feeding and changing of diapers, I had to deal with the laundry, which seemed to take forever. I used cloth diapers on both babies, and because it was a wringer washer (which everyone used in those days, by the way), it took a lot of time and energy. At least the washer my mother had when we were growing up did not have a hand-cranked wringer; a motor turned it instead.

I first had to get the coal-burning stove going in the kitchen to heat the water. It was about the size of a small kitchen table. I put a large metal tub on top and then attached a short hose to the tap to fill the tub. When the water was hot enough, which took a while, I then used a pot to transfer it into the washer.

I cranked the roller while taking each piece of clothing out of hot sudsy water and fed it through the wringer where it dropped into a big tub of cold rinse water. From there, I cranked it through the wringer one more time and it landed in a laundry basket, ready to take outside to hang on the clothesline.

With the washer set in motion, it took hours from the time of setting up to taking the clothes off the line at the end of the day to be folded. I moved from the kitchen area where I did the laundry to the small living room in the evening to finish the day's work. Since we had no living room furniture, I put Andy's crib in that room along with a little table with a basin on it. I had a chair where I'd sit to fold the clothes.

At night, I bathed Elizabeth Anne and Andy in the basin and had my own sponge bath. I considered my shower once a week at my neighbour's house a real luxury. Dougie always had his shower at the pit right after he finished his shift work. I remember one time when he happened to come home without showering for whatever reason. When he walked in the door and placed his can (a grey tin lunch box) on the table, I burst out laughing at the site of him. He still had his hard hat on with the little light attached in the front, and his face was black as coal. The whites of his eyes stood out and made his teeth look whiter than they actually were. It was so comical!

I lost any sense of time during those days because I was so busy from the time I got up in the morning to when I went to bed at night. I was always checking on Elizabeth Anne while doing the laundry, hoping the soft hum of the motor would keep her asleep a little longer so I could get her formula ready for when she woke up. I was fortunate that Andy was easy to manage and not demanding of my attention as he played by himself on the floor around my feet.

I felt very alone, though. Come to think of it, I cannot remember even one day when Dougie spent time at home with us. I already knew I was walking into a problematic situation when I decided to return to Cape Breton with him, but I never expected things to turn out this way. I also began to question why no one ever came by to see us. I concluded that I must have been doing something wrong. I thought everyone else had more worth and that I must be one of the stupidest people on this planet for the choices I had made. I was very hard on myself.

Aside from being in a relationship with someone who had no interest in being at home with me, I look back and see how I was driven by a need to prove to myself—not to anyone else—that what I did actually mattered. I became a perfectionist and tried to do everything right. I couldn't go to bed unless everything was done to my satisfaction. The house and the kids had to be clean and everything organized and ready to start again the next day. The phrase "clean freak" comes to mind. Yvonne and Justine had that reputation as well and, like them, I thought if it's worth doing, it should be done properly or not at all. This was, and still is, my way of thinking.

So every minute of each day was taken up with the preparation of formulas, feeding, bathing, changing, washing clothes and somehow trying to feed myself as well. Dougie actually got up to attend to the baby in the middle of the night a couple of times because I was so exhausted that I just didn't wake up.

One morning when I woke up feeling tired even before I had started my day, I reached out to open the venetian blind right next to our bed when I felt a hand grab my wrist from behind the thin cotton curtain on either side. It had a steel grip that made me freeze in fear, but it let go a second later. Dougie had already left for his early morning shift in the pit, and both Andy and Elizabeth Anne were still asleep. I sat up and gazed around the room, and I could hear what sounded like a child giggling.

God, am I beginning to lose my mind? I thought.

I pulled the covers over my head and decide to just stay there until one of them woke up. *I must be overdoing it as usual, I just need more rest*, I told myself. But I swear I did hear and actually feel children playing around the bottom of my bed as I fell back to sleep that morning.

That summer seemed to whizz by while I was occupied with the everyday mundane chores. I think there was only two or three times when I was able to have the car to go to Justine's place for a visit.

A couple of weeks after a visit to Justine's place, Dougie pulled into our driveway in his brother's truck. George was with him. I had no idea they were coming with the bathroom set that day. I happened to be standing next to the fence talking to our friendly neighbour. When she saw them taking the bathtub out of the truck, she pointed to the half-dug trench and said, "Dougie! Winter coming! Winter coming!" in her thick accent. I don't think I ever saw Dougie look so embarrassed as I did that day. He nodded with a sheepish grin while struggling to get the tub out of the truck. I suggested that the little room off the kitchen would be the best place to put the toilet, sink and bathtub, and they reassured me that we would soon have our much-needed bathroom. This made me very happy indeed.

As usual, I was the busy bee taking care of everything at home and hoping that Dougie would soon get busy with that unfinished trench. I was disappointed when nothing was happening, and when I brought it up it seemed to go in one ear and out the other.

The day that Justine and George paid their second visit to our place, I was in the living room where I had just finished feeding and changing Elizabeth Anne. I had her over my shoulder burping her when I spotted their car in the driveway. When I looked through the window, I saw they were standing next to the trench and obviously discussing our situation. A wave of shame came over me, and I didn't know what I was going to say to them.

As they came into the house, George pointed to Dougie's lunch can sitting on the cupboard and asked, "Where's Dougie?"

"He left for work this morning but came back saying there's no work for him today, so he was going over to Hartigan's for a while."

George looked like he wanted to say something but wasn't sure whether he should or not.

"Is that what he told you?" George asked.

Justine poked his arm and said, "Go ahead, tell her."

"What?" I asked.

"We'll, I happen to know that Dougie did have work today."

When he saw I was a little upset that Dougie had lied, he quickly changed the subject.

"I see you don't have any coal left," he said as he walked over to the stove, took the bucket and went outside to get some more.

Andy must have heard our voices because he woke up from his nap and called for me to take him out of his crib. Justine looked concerned and asked, "Where's the bathroom set?" I opened the door to the little room just off the kitchen to show her.

"What's he going to do, let it sit there and gather dust?" she asked.

"I know," I said, shaking my head. "I really don't know what I'm going to do because the ground will start to freeze very soon."

I could see Justine and George wanted to help me, but I knew there was nothing else they could do. Just to know how much they cared by what they had done already was enough to get me through the rest of that day.

That evening I confronted Dougie about his lying to me. He squirmed out of it with a few words to excuse himself, but I wasn't listening anymore. I was simply too tired. I just wanted to let it all go, and I practically fell into the bed after putting Elizabeth Anne and Andy down for the night.

Justine and George's third and final visit came only days after that. I think I was beginning to numb myself to everything. No longer "trying" to get everything right, I slowed down. I felt the weight on my shoulders, I guess. I remember sitting on a chair in the kitchen facing the stove with my feet up on the open oven door. Elizabeth Anne was in my arms drinking from her bottle, and Andy was in the living room playing with his little toy tractor when I heard Justine's low soft voice from behind.

"Can I come in?"

"Oh! You surprised me! I didn't know you were coming," I said, propping Elizabeth Anne over my shoulder.

"How are you making out?" she said with a smile.

"Nothing is happening, as you can see, and complaining doesn't make it any better."

"Where's Dougie?" George asked as he came in behind Justine.

"I don't know, and I don't care," I said in a discouraged tone.

"Well, we can't stay. We just came from shopping and stopped by to see how you're doing," Justine said, her smile changing to a rather worried look. "We bought something for you while we were shopping just now. You want to bring it in, George?" she asked.

As he went out the door, she reached out and took my hand, placing what felt like a piece of paper inside and clasping her other hand over it.

"Here, this is for you."

I opened my hand to see a fifty dollar bill!

"What?" I said, surprised and somewhat confused.

Just then George came through the door carrying what looked like a trunk.

"Maybe you'll be able to make use of this," he said with a kind but serious look on his face.

I was really confused and didn't have a clue as to what was happening.

"We better get back," he said. "My mother is babysitting Patrick for us, and I told her we wouldn't be long."

They left in a rather hurried manner, and as I followed them to their car, I tried to find some words to express my gratitude, but all that came out was a meek, "Thank you so much."

Then Justine said, "You could put the trunk at the bottom of your bed if you'd like and put all your blankets inside like I did with the cedar chest George gave me when we were engaged."

"Yes, I remember. It gave the clothes that nice cedar smell."

Waving goodbye, I noticed how much their visit had perked me up. I got right back to feeding Elizabeth Anne, but I wondered why they bought me that trunk and gave me money. As I said, my mind had been in a numb-like state and I really was having trouble with clarity of mind. Slowly it dawned on me that they were simply showing some support should things go from bad to worse between Dougie and I. It actually opened my eyes to the urgency of my situation with the cold weather just around the corner.

Anita and I had been out of touch with each other ever since she gave birth to her son Torbin, which was only a couple of weeks after Andy was born. Both were now eighteen months old, and Elizabeth Anne was four months. So I thought I'd find out how things were going for Anita and Chris.

I contacted her to see if she'd be open to me coming over to Toronto for a visit. This issue of having no bathroom with winter approaching had consumed my mind to the point that, I must admit, I would have gone anywhere just to get away for a while. I had no idea how they were doing. I only knew that they were living in the same apartment building as our sister Yvonne in Toronto.

So Anita agreed that I shouldn't stay with the way things were in New Waterford. Elizabeth Anne and I could sleep on a blow-up mattress they had in storage, and Andy could use the cot that was in Torbin's bedroom next to his crib. I told her we'd probably be there in about a week's time.

Meanwhile I didn't want to tell Dougie about the money Justine gave me or the fact that I intended to go away for a while. This bothered me quite a bit because I'm always so upfront with whatever I am doing. Anyway, I started to prepare by putting a couple of things into the trunk. Dougie and I were not the type to argue or fight with each other, but I was still on edge that I might have a problem if I let him know about my plan. I know he didn't like it when Justine and George gave me that trunk, and I sensed he was a little suspicious lately. However, something had to drastically change for me to stay because it was November and the ground was about to start freezing.

When Dougie walked in unexpectedly with his friend to get something he needed, I had the trunk open in front of me putting some baby clothes and diapers in that I had washed the day before.

"What are you doing?" he asked.

"I'm putting some clothes together for a trip to Toronto because I want to visit Anita for a while."

He just walked away saying, "Come on, let's go," to his friend. Because he didn't let me know what he was thinking, I was beginning to get a bit nervous. Maybe fifteen minutes or so went by when I heard a car door close outside. I was attending to Elizabeth Anne and figured it must be Dougie. As I came into the kitchen carrying Elizabeth Anne, I was taken aback to see Olga, Dougie's sister, come through the back door. A tall, heavy-set woman, she was a bit intimidating when she stepped into the kitchen with her arms crossed as if ready for an argument.

"I hope you don't think you're taking Andy with you," she said in a threatening manner. "That's Dougie's little man!"

I didn't know what to think or say, so I just ignored her while getting Elizabeth Anne's bottle ready. *Why would she suddenly show up in this defensive mode?* I thought. Then it dawned on me that Dougie must have gone to his family and told them I was leaving. Maybe he was afraid I might take both kids with me (which I intended to do).

"Well, okay, if Dougie doesn't want Andy to come with me, then he can stay. No problem," I said.

"When are you leaving?" she asked, her tone and demeanour becoming less defensive.

"I planned to go next week, but I changed my mind and want to go now if I can, in case Dougie tries to stop me from taking Elizabeth Anne with me."

She seemed annoyed by my determination to leave right away.

"I'll take Andy back with me now then," she said, "and I'll ask Ewen if he'll drive you to the train station in Sydney."

I wasn't sure whether or not to believe what Olga said, but I gathered everything at the door anyway to be ready to go. It seemed like only minutes went by before Ewen showed up offering to drive me to Sydney to get the train. I always thought his whole family was against me, so I really didn't expect they would be willing to help me that day. Anyway, we made it to the train station just in time.

As I was getting settled into my seat with Elizabeth Anne, I couldn't believe my eyes when I saw Dougie come running alongside the train. He hopped on and rushed down the aisle to where I was sitting. I was too stunned to speak as he reached down and tried to take Elizabeth Anne out of my arms.

"Leave her here! you don't have to take her with you!" he said trying to keep his voice down.

"NO!... NO!.. she's coming with ME!" I insisted - desperately hanging onto her.

Just then the train suddenly jolted and the words ALL ABOARD! rang out throwing me into a panic.

At that moment he reluctantly let go, turned and quickly walked back to the exit where the conductor was patiently standing by. I fought back the tears as the train slowly started to pull away. Then on my way to the counter to have her bottle filled with milk, I overheard a couple of passengers commenting on what they had just witnessed, and couldn't help but feel the shame. I really don't remember anything else after that terrible episode.

Chapter 10

The next memory I have is being with Anita, Chris and Torbin in their apartment in Toronto.

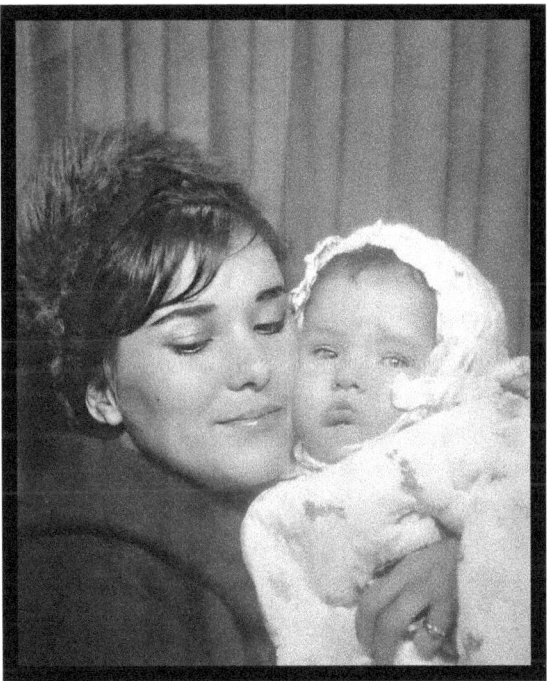

Anna and baby Liz

I happened to be in Yvonne's apartment the next day when I heard a little knock on the door. It was Anita. She wanted me to come and help her with something. I don't remember what it was, but I happened to be holding Elizabeth Anne in my arms at the time. I turned to Mama, who was sitting at the kitchen table, and asked, "Would you mind holding her for a few minutes?" She got up, started walking towards her bedroom and said, "Just prop her up with some pillows there on the couch." Her response hurt, and when I mentioned it to Anita as we walked back to her apartment she said, "I'm not surprised, she has never held Torbin either. Guess she just doesn't like babies."

"Oh God, don't remind me," I said half-jokingly but feeling the underlying pain at the same time.

I was there about a week and a half when I began to have serious thoughts about where I would spend the winter. That's when the crying spells started. Yvonne was concerned and suggested I seek professional help for my state of mind. She even arranged an appointment for me to see a doctor, but I didn't go.

Afterwards, Anita said she was told that if I return to that same situation in New Waterford, I could very well have a mental breakdown and never come out of it. Yvonne suggested I go to Montreal and stay with Tony temporarily; she thought it might be okay since he and Rosemary had recently separated. *Maybe I could babysit his little girl while he's at work, and this way I could keep Elizabeth Anne with me*, I thought. This seemed like a good solution, so I decided to go to Montreal if Tony would agree, which he did. Yvonne gave me one of her own suitcases and advised me to leave my trunk at Anita's place for the time being.

When Tony picked me up at the train station, I wasn't sure if he was open to me being there even though he agreed over the phone to give it a try. After a couple of days I was afraid it might not work out because his three-year-old girl was so hyperactive; I was used to Andy and Elizabeth Anne who were the complete opposite. I was having trouble sleeping, worrying about how all this was going to turn out.

One day when Elizabeth Anne was asleep, I dozed off on the couch while Tony's daughter was colouring. When Tony came home from work, he was furious with me.

"Look at the walls! They're marked up with crayon! You can't let her do that!"

He was right, of course, and I felt terrible about what happened. I went into the bathroom to shower hoping he would calm down. When I came out, he had my suitcase packed and at the door. While putting his jacket on, he said, "Get the baby ready, you can't stay here."

"But where are we going?" I asked.

"You'll see soon enough," he said, still angry at me.

We drove about ten minutes before he pulled up in front of an apartment building. He got out and handed me my suitcase as I struggled to hold onto Elizabeth Anne while getting out of the car.

"So where are we going?" I asked, by now totally confused.

He didn't answer as I followed him to the entrance. Then as he put my suitcase down in front of the door he said, "Don't you dare tell him I drove you here!"

"What? Who?" I asked.

"Jimmy," he replied as he quickly turned and walked back to his car. "Tell him you took the bus!"

Oh my God, NO! He took me to Jimmy's place! I looked at the names on the wall in the entrance and saw his name. I almost fainted. The next thing I remember is standing at his door.

"What the hell are you doing here? Tony brought you over, didn't he?"

Elizabeth Anne started to squirm as I was holding her. I started to tremble then broke down. Suddenly I felt the sting of a slap across my face.

"Don't get hysterical here!" he said in a commanding voice. "These are bachelor apartments—no kids are allowed!"

Elizabeth Anne started to cry and I was losing my grip on her as I turned to leave.

"You made your bed, now lie in it!" he said in a mocking tone as he plunked my suitcase down in the hallway and slammed the door.

I picked it up and ran out to the sidewalk in hysterics. *This is not really happening!* I told myself. My mind was reeling when I suddenly discovered I was lost. Tears streaming down my face, I kept on walking until I came to an intersection.

"Thank God," I said when I saw a bus shelter.

I sat down inside. Poor Elizabeth Anne kept crying off and on—it was past her feeding time. I sat there trying to figure out my next move and concluded I would have to go back to Tony's place as the bus pulled up in front of me. I stepped inside trying to hold onto both the suitcase and Elizabeth Anne. As the driver slowly pulled away, I asked rather timidly, "Can I get to the l'Acadie Estates Apartments from here?"

"Yes, but you'll have to transfer to another bus a few streets from here; I'll let you know when."

I stepped off the bus in front of the building where Tony lived, knowing full well that he would be furious with me for coming back. *If I could just stay the night at least, then I can go back to Toronto tomorrow,* I told myself. Once inside the lobby, I sat in the lounge chair to get Elizabeth Anne's pablum and bottle out of her bunting bag so I could feed her right away. But the more I thought about how Tony would react to my coming back, the more frightened I became. I tried to come up with some other solution, like maybe work in a house where I could keep Elizabeth Anne with me? But tonight I needed to stay there.

When I walked towards his door, I must have had some kind of a panic attack similar to the one I had on the train when Doug tried to take Elizabeth Anne from me. *NO! I can't!* I told myself as I raised my hand to knock. *God help me, I don't know what to do!* I turned and kept walking down the hallway not knowing where I was going. I opened the door at the end, entered the stairwell and somehow ended up on the next floor. *This is crazy, I know, but I'm going to knock on one of these doors*, I told myself. When I did, a tall, blond, middle-aged woman wearing lots of make-up and a lovely lounge outfit opened it.

"Yes?" she said in a friendly voice.

"Can I come inside for a minute?" I asked.

"Sure, who are you looking for?"

I saw immediately that she was a kind and friendly person, so I explained my situation and asked if she might have the newspaper so I could look in the domestic help wanted section. She picked up the *Montreal Gazette* and started skimming, saying it just might be possible to work in a home where I can keep Elizabeth Anne with me. After a few calls without any luck, she suggested I call back the one needing someone to start right away as a live-in.

"But first I want to talk to a friend of mine," she said.

She then called a friend and explained my situation as I waited patiently. Her call ended with a smile and "Thank you so much!" while giving me the thumbs up sign. She was so positive about everything that my hopes jumped sky-high. She reassured me that there was a wonderful family who would be happy to look after Elizabeth Anne for me while I was working as a live-in domestic.

"So don't worry, just call that number I circled on the paper and let them know you will be there tonight."

The lady whom I had already spoken to on the phone recognized my voice and said I could come anytime, no problem. Her address happened to be in the upper class neighbourhood of Mount Royal, and we arrived on their doorstep shortly after our phone call. I left my luggage there saying I would be back as soon as we placed Elizabeth Anne with a family not far away in the suburb of Ville Saint-Laurent.

I was ever so grateful to that lady for being so kind, helping me with the right connections and driving me to where I needed to go.

When we arrived at Pilon's, the French-speaking family's home in Saint-Laurent, they welcomed us with open arms. They took Elizabeth Anne while showing us a nice little bedroom she could use, and I was reassured that she would be in good hands. I was told they took in foster children once in a while to help out until the parents were in a better position to care for them. There couldn't have been a better solution, and I thanked God over and over in my mind as we arrived back in Mount Royal where I would live and start working the very next day.

The people who hired me were polite but not that friendly. They told me exactly what my duties were and that I was to keep to myself in the tiny apartment-like space I'd have in the basement of their giant mansion. I was given a black cotton uniform with a little white apron to wear while working during the day.

I found my way to Elizabeth Anne by bus a few days later. I then visited on a regular basis on weekends. She seemed to be doing just fine with them, so I was glad about that, but I missed Andy a lot. I kept to myself and focused only on getting by as best I could under the circumstances.

Chapter 11

Eight months after I took Elizabeth Anne and left New Waterford, she turned one year old while living with the Pilon family. They were kind and took good care of her. Andy had his second birthday in June while living with Dougie's family back in New Waterford. It bothered me that they were not together or even with me, but I didn't understand how to fix the situation.

I began to have terrible nightmares at least once a month where I'd find myself lost and totally helpless in a large city. Sometimes it was in Montreal and other times in different cities in other parts of the world. But wherever it happened, I was always in the exact same predicament.

It began with me walking along a busy street when suddenly I'd lose my way as I turned onto a side street. Realizing I was lost, I'd turn to strangers passing by to ask for directions, but they all ignored me as if I wasn't there. I'd keep on walking in the dream that seemed to go on forever, and when I did finally wake up, I felt totally exhausted and discouraged. I always managed to rise above it and get on with my day, and these nightmares came on less over the years, resurfacing only when I was faced with stressful situations.

Anita called me out of the blue one day saying she was coming to Montreal with Torbin for a visit. When she saw the place where Elizabeth Anne was living, she wanted to put Torbin in that home also. I didn't know what to make of her decision—was she breaking up with Chris or what? She didn't share what was going on in their relationship, but I was happy for her that the family agreed to take Torbin in.

A couple of weeks later, Chris arrived from Toronto. There didn't seem to be any problem between them, so I wondered why Anita wanted to place Torbin with that family. The Pilons seemed to like Chris a lot, which was good. He was polite and could be quite charming when he flashed his big friendly smile. So when he came to take Torbin out one day without Anita knowing that he was coming, they thought it would be okay. But when he didn't return that evening with Torbin as promised, they became worried and told Anita what happened.

She, of course, was shocked. She called Yvonne, but he was not there either! She returned to Toronto immediately to find that Chris and Torbin had disappeared altogether. It appeared he had abducted Torbin and possibly went back to Denmark where he had lived before coming to Canada. I felt so bad for Anita, and she didn't seem the same after that awful experience. I tried to get through to her, but she wouldn't open up. It was as if the pain was too deep.

I recalled a few moments right after our double ring ceremony when she appeared to want to tell me something but just didn't know how to say it. When I asked what was wrong, she let me know—in a roundabout way— that she thought he might be gay and only wanted to marry her because he wanted a child. She never said a word about her suspicion after that, so I just assumed there was no problem after all. They seemed to be getting along just fine whenever I was with them.

After Chris abducted their son and disappeared without a trace that summer, Dougie suddenly showed up in Montreal. He brought Andy with him and rented a room for the short time he said he planned to stay. I left the home in Mount Royal, took Elizabeth Anne out of the Pilon's home and moved in with Dougie. He soon made it clear that he was going to take both kids back to Cape Breton with him. He said things had improved back home and I was to go back with him.

I was torn between putting Elizabeth Anne back into the home and going back to working as a domestic or taking another chance and returning to New Waterford to try to make us work. After a heated argument over what to do, I decided to stay in Montreal. But Dougie was relentless; there was no way he was going to leave without Elizabeth Anne, and I could see that.

In a heated moment, he punched me in the left shoulder, which caused me to let go of her and he grasped her out of my arms. She started to cry, and I instinctively ran out the door and around the corner to the police station where I begged for help. There were two officers, one in uniform and one in a suit, and he drove me back in an unmarked car. When we arrived, Dougie was walking towards his car carrying Elizabeth Anne and Andy was already inside.

"Don't let him take her! I want to keep her here with me!" I shouted, running alongside the police officer as he approached Dougie's car.

"Okay, calm down. I want to know who's the provider?"

"I am!" Dougie replied.

"I'm sorry but I can't do anything, madam. You'll need a lawyer."

At that point, Dougie slowly pulled away, leaving me standing there with my mouth open in disbelief.

The officer opened the door to his car and said, "Come on, get in." He suggested we go for a little drive up to Mount Royal a few blocks away to "calm down." Everything seemed so unreal. When he came to a stop on the mountain, he just sat there not saying a word and I began to feel uneasy, so I got out of the car and went over to the lookout.

There was nobody else around. I started to think I shouldn't have gone up there, so I walked back to the car. When I opened the door, I was stunned to see him sitting there staring at me with his pants open, exposing himself. I quickly slammed the door shut and ran back to the lookout. I didn't know what to do next. *How dare he!* I automatically assumed because he was a police officer that I'd be safe with him! I returned to the car, slowly opened the door and got back in with my right hand firmly holding onto the door handle, ready to jump out should it be necessary. I was trying to hold it together, to think clearly enough to get back safely.

Suddenly he reached over and stuffed a five dollar bill into a side pocket on my purse and started the car. *Why did he do that? Please let him take me straight back to my place,* I prayed. And thank God he did. By now I couldn't wait to get back into our room where I wanted to be alone and just cry my eyes out, which I did until I fell asleep.

I was awakened suddenly by the sound of someone unlocking the door. I held my breath, unable to move in fear. Then I sighed in relief and exhaled when I saw who it was.

"Dougie! Oh my God! It's YOU! I thought you had left already!"

"No, I went to get someone to help me with the drive back to New Waterford. He's waiting in the car with the kids, so we're leaving now. You shouldn't have called the cops! They can't stop me from taking my own kids back home with me!"

I almost blurted out what had happened while he was gone, but I caught myself because it would make the situation even worse.

"Okay maybe I should go back with you and give it another try," I said.

That sudden change from my side helped reduce the tension so that I was able to think clearly enough to quickly pack my things to leave.

We started out with Dougie at the wheel, me in the passenger seat and Elizabeth Anne in the middle. Martin from New Waterford came along to help with the driving, and he was in the back seat with Andy. After the first half of the trip, we stopped for a bite to eat and Dougie and Martin switched spots.

It was around five o'clock in the evening when we were back on the road again, driving through Quebec. Everyone was quiet and beginning to feel a little tired after so many hours on the road. I was dozing while holding

Elizabeth Anne on my lap when Dougie yelled, "JE-SUS!" My eyes popped wide open in time to catch a glimpse of a farmer's tractor turning around in a circle in the middle of the highway as we started to descend the hill. It was directly in our path but quickly swerved to the left at the same time as our car swerved to the right trying to avoid a collision.

We slammed head-on into the tractor!

In that split second before we hit, I instinctively leaned over Elizabeth Anne, twisting my body to shield her. I felt the impact of the steering wheel against my spine and must have passed out, because the next thing I remember is someone shaking me and asking if I was okay. All of us were in shock, of course. Dougie jumped out from the back of the car and pulled at Martin.

"Come on, get out—You don't have a driver's licence! Make sure you say I was the one driving if anybody asks," he said.

Just then a car with a Nova Scotia licence plate slowed down and pulled off the highway. A man got out and came rushing over to see if he could help. He said he and his wife were on their way home to Halifax and asked where we were headed. When I told them I have a sister who lived in Dartmouth near Halifax they offered to take me there since it was on their way. Decisions were quickly made within those few minutes while waiting for help to arrive. Dougie said our car would have to be scrapped, so he and Martin would take the train back with Elizabeth Anne and Andy.

"You can get in the car with them," he said. "They'll take you to your sister's place."

We seemed to drive forever. I know they stopped a couple of times because they said I should go to the washroom. But I was in a weird numb-like state and refused to move. It's strange now that I think about it, but whenever I experienced trauma over the years, I was able to vividly recall not only the incident but the details for a long time afterwards. Once in a while, though—like right now as I am trying to remember what happened when I arrived back in New Waterford after the car accident—nothing surfaces.

Maybe I should mention here how the idea of writing a book came about in the first place. After living through a number of traumatic experiences after Dougie and I finally split up, I was fortunate enough to undergo three years of therapy with a wonderful psychotherapist. During one of our sessions she said she wanted to have a psychiatrist come in and sit with us for an hour. She wanted to know if I would need medication and if so, what should be prescribed.

When the hour was up, the psychiatrist suggested I take some pills to help get me through that particular rough period. What stands out in my mind about that day was the comment he made as he was getting up to leave.

"You know … you could write a book."

When I sort of laughed in response, he leaned forward and said, "I'm serious." I never forgot the way he looked me straight in the eye with such conviction when he said it. Of course, at that time I would not have been able to write about my experiences since the memories were still fresh and painful. But many years later, I'm finally able to recall and write about my past without feeling much of the mental and emotional pain that was associated with it.

Back to 1964 just after our car crash. When I went back home and saw that the sewer pipe still wasn't in the trench, I must have freaked out, because I decided to go right back to Montreal. There was absolutely no doubt left in my mind that this was not going to work out because nothing had changed for the better. The same non-communication with his family and only promises from him that all would work out left me terribly disappointed to say the least.

It became clear that I should not uproot Elizabeth Anne again by placing her in yet another unpredictable situation. So with the understanding that both her and Andy's need to have a stable home was more important than my wanting to have them with me, I made the heart-wrenching decision to leave them with Dougie and his family.

Back in Montreal, I found a room on the same street where Dougie had rented a place. I had no idea what I was going to do, but I knew I had to leave when I did or else I was going to lose my mind altogether.

A few days later I had a reality check when I realized it was the end of September and I did not get my period on the twenty-fifth. I told myself it was due to all the stress I had just been through, but by the end of the month I was certain I was pregnant again. I became distraught and couldn't sleep. *What am I supposed to do now?* kept repeating in my mind.

When I called Dougie to give him the news, he was surprised but didn't seem to be upset about it. He just told me I should come back home again. I was confused and felt like my life was just going in circles!

Shortly afterwards I was walking on the street near my place when who came walking around the corner but Dougie! Mixed emotions welled up inside as we approached each other. I didn't know what to expect. As you've likely come to discover, he had a tendency to take action without discussing it with me first, and this was one of those times. I had no idea he had any intention of coming to Montreal again.

So here he was out of the blue saying he had just rented a furnished one-bedroom apartment on Hope Street just around the corner from me. I moved in with him, all the while wondering just what he had in mind. When I told him I was not about to go back to New Waterford—pregnant or not—he said he was going to apply for work at the construction site of Place Victoria, an office tower in downtown Montreal. He had maintained connections with his New Waterford buddies and they always helped each other out. Word got around that there was a need for workers to help install huge glass windows in the office tower, so Dougie got in touch with the general foreman, who was also from Cape Breton, and he was hired immediately.

Even though he seemed to adjust quickly in his new job and was making a good salary, Dougie and I had not made any progress as far as our relationship was concerned. It didn't bother me when he spent time out with his friends when not working. However, there was one time when he came home drunk around three o'clock in the morning carrying a small portable TV. He told me that a couple of "queers," as he called them, tried to connect with him at the bar, so he pretended to be interested. Then he said he went with one of them to his apartment and "beat the living daylights out of him."

"Got myself a TV while I was at it," he said with a grin.

We often clashed over his unacceptable actions, and this was no different.

"You are lucky you didn't get caught and thrown in jail!" I said.

To this day I feel so sorry for whomever the victim was.

Dougie continued work on Place Victoria while bringing in a good salary. He sent money back home to his family who were taking very good care of Andy and Elizabeth Anne, which gave me some comfort.

Their family obviously had a bond that for some reason I was never able to feel a part of. At times when I felt disconnected and alone, I would be overcome with a desire to go somewhere—anywhere—where I thought I might find some acceptance. It was difficult for me to face the reality that running away got me nowhere. I only ended up alone in a city that I hated. Despite this fact, I still could not bring myself to even think about going back to New Waterford again. I did not know which way to turn.

On May 28, 1965, I woke up after a restless night with what I instinctively knew was my first contraction. It was just after 5 a.m. Knowing labour had started, I woke Dougie and immediately got into the shower. My suitcase was ready next to the bed. Just before I stepped out of the shower, I felt a tremendous gush of water and realized that my water broke! This was the first time I had experienced this, so I felt a little nervous, but it wasn't long before I was safe and sound in the delivery room.

The labour was not like the previous ones at all. It was what is called a dry birth. I remember having a difficult time with the painful contractions that seemed to be more intense and painful than when I had Andy and

Elizabeth Anne. They say every birth is different, and this was true for me. Finally, Lynn Marie, a name I picked out of a book of baby names there in the hospital, made her appearance. I was so happy she was healthy, with all fingers and toes in the right place, and that all went well for us. I do not recall Dougie being there with me in the hospital, but he did come to get us when it was time for me to leave at least.

A few weeks later, Dougie was gone for a whole day, which was unusual, and I became worried. When he wasn't at work, he was often either at his friend's place or at a bar called the Cozy Club around the corner on Saint-Catherine Street. There were no cell phones at that time, and we never kept in touch when he went out.

When he finally came home, I became scared and upset when he confessed that he spent the day making arrangements to go back east. He hadn't said a word to me about it. He said he gave his notice at Place Victoria and that one of his buddies and his girlfriend were ready to go back with him.

"And you're coming too!" he announced.

That was the spark that ignited the fire. I laid awake that night wondering if I could keep Lynn with me and knowing full well it would not be the best thing for her. Dougie wanted to leave first thing in the morning and was pushing me to get everything together to go, but I resisted up to the last minute. When his friends arrived early the next morning, I panicked.

"I am not going back to New Waterford!" I said. "And Lynn is staying here with me."

Dougie stepped in and picked her up, saying, "Okay, let's go!"

I totally freaked out as he quickly walked to the car with me running behind. Sound familiar? This time I didn't run to a police station. I calmly strode back to our apartment and grabbed a kitchen knife.

"I'll kill you!" I screamed, running at him.

I didn't mean it, of course, and it accomplished nothing in the long run. It just made everyone feel sorry for him when he returned home. He told his family that I was crazy and that I tried to kill him. GOD! I honestly believe I was temporarily insane, and the effects of that episode lasted for many days after he left. I became depressed to the point of thinking about ending my life, but when I seriously began having such thoughts, I managed to pull myself together somehow.

When I called Anita, she told me she didn't know how to cope with life either. So there she was in Toronto without Torbin, and there I was in Montreal without Andy, Elizabeth Anne and now Lynn, who was only six weeks old. During our short conversation, Anita said she had gotten in touch with our brother Louis (the one who brought the two sets of dolls home many years ago), and she gave me his telephone number. She told me he was living in Montreal, but that was all she knew.

I called and shared my story with him and he decided we should get together. I asked if he would like to come over but he said he couldn't because he didn't have a vehicle and it would take too long by bus.

"I had a car accident and was badly injured many years ago," he said. "I have not been behind the wheel since."

"That's okay, I will come over to your place then," I said.

A few days later when I dropped by, I expected he'd be alone, but he had a friend with him. He introduced him as Andy, said he was also from New Waterford and that he was Dougie's boss at the Place Victoria. They were both very understanding of my plight. It wasn't as if I wanted their sympathy—I had only mentioned the basic facts, I didn't go on about it.

I thought we had a rather pleasant visit that day, and I wanted to stay in touch since I was totally alone in Montreal. There was no way I was going to get in touch with Tony or Jimmy again, that's for sure. As Andy was going out the door, he handed me a piece of paper with his name and number on it, saying, "If you need anything just give me a call." After he left, Louis told me Andy had separated from his wife about six months ago.

She apparently went to live with her mother in Toronto, taking their two children with her. We were obviously going through similar experiences, so I kept his phone number just in case I might want to talk to him again.

The apartment that Dougie and I had was about to be rented to someone else, so I knew I'd have to look for another place to live. I went through the ads to see if I could find a place to work in a home and quickly found a live-in domestic position once again. This time it was with an elderly couple who had their own chauffeur. I was given a decent room downstairs in their home, and I did not have to wear a uniform, which I preferred. They showed more respect towards me than the previous place, so I felt OK about the job; it was the only alternative to going back to New Waterford.

I missed the kids a lot but did not know what to do about the situation. My hands were tied, but I realized time was passing quickly and they might forget about me altogether. I decided to contact Louis's friend Andy about a month after our first introduction. We had a rather long conversation and we got together that weekend for lunch. I was comfortable with our meeting as we mainly talked about how we wanted to be with our kids but were unable to find solutions to our ongoing relationship problems. I think we both just needed to talk to someone about what we were going through. We had no problem sharing our stories and decided to meet again the following week.

It was autumn, and it was hard to believe how much had happened in the past year. I had become pregnant and had given birth to baby Lynn who was now living with Dougie and his family back in New Waterford. I spent some time reflecting on what had taken place and wondering if the choices I made were the right ones. I still wasn't sure about my next move and where it might lead.

Andy and I began to spend weekends together, and it seemed to be a temporary solution for both of us. But we were lonely for our kids and we had no idea how we were going to solve our relationship problems. It's not that Andy and I were "in love" with each other but more like we kind of needed someone to turn to at that point in time. Living alone in the city was not working out for either of us.

Nineteen sixty-four had come and gone with so much drama that I could barely think straight. The traumatic situations were all just too much. I was left in such a state of uncertainty that I began to doubt my own sanity. *Why am I making so many decisions where I end up in even more problematic situations? Why do I always run away when unable to cope?*

To start off 1965, I was faced with yet another dilemma when I discovered I was pregnant again! I was beside myself with guilt. *How I could I have let this happen?* I already had three children with Dougie and now I was pregnant with Andy's baby! I felt terrible! I couldn't even bring myself to tell him at first. I was too busy beating myself up for being careless. My inner dialogue was a repeating record of *There must be something seriously wrong with me!* I began to think I really did need professional help.

Andy noticed a change in me the next weekend when we met and wondered why I wasn't open to communicating with him. I wasn't able to bring up the pregnancy because I was just trying to figure out what in the world I would do about it. I knew I should talk to a professional, but instead I just kept it all to myself.

Two and a half months went by before I told Andy. We were sitting outside on his balcony catching the last rays of the evening sun, both of us in a rather quiet mood. I was ready to accept whatever reaction he would have to the news, and I hoped I would do the right thing to find a solution.

"There is something I have to tell you, Andy. Something I know I should have told you a couple of months ago," I said.

He sat there with an inquisitive look and said, "What is it?"

"Well, it is not something I wanted to have happen, and when I found out I was unable to say anything about it because I was just too upset."

He leaned forward with a more serious expression.

"What happened? It's okay, you can tell me," he said.

"Yes, but I'm having a hard time coming out with it. I don't know how you are going to take it—that's why it took me this long to bring it up."

"Aw, come on, it can't be that bad, what happened?"

I paused for a moment, then slowly each word came out almost in a whisper.

"I … I am … pregnant."

His eyes opened wide, and he just sat there staring at me.

"Are you sure?"

"Oh, I'm sure all right. I'm almost three months along now. I know I should have let you know right away, but I just couldn't bring myself to tell you."

"Have you decided what you are going to do?" he asked with a worried look on his face.

"There is no way I will be able to keep this baby! I just gave birth to Lynn Marie in May!"

The seriousness of our situation weighed heavily on our shoulders as we discussed the options for another hour or so.

"I'm so overwhelmed by everything that's been happening this past year, and I know I brought it all onto myself!" I said as I got up to leave. "And I'm not sure how long I will be able to continue working in this condition."

"Does anyone else know you're pregnant?"

"No. The couple I work for have no idea, but I'm afraid they will know soon enough."

The next day, Andy stopped in to talk to me. I led him into the sun porch where I figured he wanted to continue our conversation regarding our current situation. I expected there would be a little tension between us now that he knew the predicament we were in, but I was surprised to see how nervous he seemed to be.

"I'm not sure where to begin," he said with a sort of apologetic tone.

"It's okay," I said. "I know it was quite a shock when I told you the news yesterday about—"

"I have to tell you what happened after you left my place last night."

"Oh? Something happened?"

"Yes, I was getting ready for bed when I heard voices coming from outside my apartment door. When I went to investigate, the door opened and my daughter came running towards me yelling, 'Daddy! We're home!' I was shocked! Believe me I had absolutely no idea they were coming back last night—none!"

"Oh my God! What if they had arrived earlier when we were sitting there talking about the predicament that you and I are in right now! Or even worse, when I stayed over Saturday night!"

"I don't want to even think about it," he said. "The reason I'm here is to ask that you be careful not to call me, okay? I'll get back to you tomorrow at noon, I really have to go now."

I was on edge the next day waiting for this call, and the phone rang at noon. It was Andy.

"I was talking to a buddy of mine who had a similar problem a few years ago, and he told me how they solved it. I can tell you about it tomorrow. I'll come by to pick you up around seven o'clock, okay?"

I agreed but could hardly get to sleep that night wondering what he might have in mind. I wasn't able to make a decision on my own, and I wanted to believe he could help me somehow—that maybe, just maybe, there might be a solution to our dilemma after all.

He arrived the next evening with an anxious look on his face.

"We will be going to a motel close by," he said, "because it's the only place I can think of right now, if you don't mind."

"That's okay," I replied.

I needed more information, and by now I was afraid of what laid ahead for both of us.

We had a serious conversation covering everything from how we got into this relationship in the first place to how I must decide what would be best regarding my pregnancy. When I told him I felt the best thing would be for me to give the baby up for adoption, he said, "Well, there is another option my friend told me about that could work as well."

"What do you mean?" I asked.

He took a small package out of his pocket and opened it to reveal two small purple pills.

"This is what he gave to his girlfriend, and it worked."

"What do you mean, 'it worked'?"

"If you use these pills before you're in your third month, it will abort the fetus," he said.

"I really don't know what to do," I said, on the verge of tears.

"All right, we'll leave it for now. I just wanted to explain everything and leave it up to you."

He opened a little overnight bag and took out a couple of things.

"I brought this in case you decide to use these pills, okay?"

"What did you bring?"

"I was told this is what we would need."

After going back and forth over my options for I don't know how long, I made the painful decision to go ahead and use the pills. He took towels and a rain coat out of the bag and placed them on the bed, saying I had to lie down because the pills had to be inserted into the vagina. We would then have to wait for the pills to work. When I started to bleed, I would have to sit on the toilet and wait. Which I did. It was only a matter of minutes before I felt a strong burning sensation along with a lot of bleeding, which made me really, really scared.

"Oh my God! What am I doing?!"

I started to cry. Suddenly, with a little push out came what looked like a small blob of thick blood.

"It's burning too much! I need to lie down!"

"The raincoat that's under the towels will protect the mattress. You will have to stay there until the bleeding stops," he said.

Thankfully, the bleeding did stop within a matter of minutes, but I couldn't stop crying. The feeling of guilt was overwhelming. Andy tried to console me but to no avail.

"I can't believe this is happening," I moaned. "Please just take me back. I want to get out of here."

"But we shouldn't go anywhere until there is no more bleeding," he said.

It was another couple of hours before we left the motel, both of us feeling awful, to say the least. Andy came downstairs with me to my room and helped me get into bed. He tried his best to reassure me that everything would be okay. He took the stained towels out of his bag and put them in a pail of water to be washed the next day. I had to wear a pad as if I were menstruating. It was like I was in the middle of a nightmare that I couldn't wake up from.

After doing the laundry, I spent the entire day in bed going over and over in my mind what happened. I honestly felt I was on the verge of a having a serious mental breakdown.

Chapter 12

I decided to make an appointment with a doctor a few days later. I explained what happened, and he told me he'd have to examine me to see what damage had been done.

"Well, I can tell you one thing for certain, you are still pregnant. The sack the baby is in has not been punctured. Those pills badly burned the lining of the vagina, causing a chunk to come out which you mistook for the fetus."

I was immediately relieved to know I would still be able to bring this pregnancy to full term. I couldn't believe that I had actually considered aborting, let alone going through with it. I must say I still feel a pang of guilt to this day whenever I think about it.

I had not heard from Andy since that night, but for some reason I felt the need to let him know the result of my doctor's visit, even though I knew we would not be seeing each other again. I asked Louis to ask Andy to please give me a call, which he did a few days later.

Andy was clearly feeling the guilt, too, and he didn't know what to say when I gave him the news. That phone call was the last time we ever spoke to each other. When I talked to Louis again a few weeks later, he told me what was happening with Andy.

"There's something Andy didn't tell you, so I will, since you're not seeing each other anymore."

"Oh really? Something I didn't know?"

"Yes, he told me that his wife came back because she wanted her baby to be born in Ottawa, not Toronto."

"What are you talking about? You mean she's pregnant?"

"Yes, she's due in a couple of weeks from now."

"Oh my God! This is getting to be more unbelievable with each passing day! I will need some time to process this, it's just too much to take in right now."

I spent the next few months trying to accept the consequences of our actions, all the while hoping I will be strong enough to face whatever laid ahead.

I was seven and a half months along when I noticed a blood stain on my underwear and began to get worried. When I mentioned it, the lady I worked for also became concerned. But I did not expect the reaction from both her and her husband when they sat down with me the next day to talk about my condition. They let me know in a caring manner that they were afraid I could end up having a premature birth if I continued working and said they would have to find a replacement for me over the weekend.

My mind jumped into overdrive trying to figure out what I should do to get through the weeks ahead. I can't remember ever really thinking through problems I had to face as one would normally do. I guess that's why I always ended up stuck in situations like the one I was in.

I suddenly felt desperate to connect with someone—anyone—who might be able to help. I got my little address book out, but it only had the family's numbers and Andy's. There was a tiny piece of paper stuck inside the pages that had only a telephone number on it. *Who could that be?* I thought. I was curious, so I called, but there was no answer. In the bottom of my purse, I found a business card from a photographer who used to live next door to Dougie and I who worked for the *Montreal Gazette*. He loved working with the camera and offered to take some pictures of us sometime. He was an older man in his mid-fifties with a strong Danish accent. A decent, polite person named Steve. I remember him showing us a large black and white shot he had taken of the Mercier Bridge in Montreal at night. *That's when he must have given me his business card*, I thought.

I had no one else to connect with, so I dialed Steve's number. I didn't say much, just mentioned that I found his business card and wondered how he was doing and if I might drop by. He sounded happy to hear from me and gave me his new address, so I found my way by bus the next day. He was quite surprised to see me in my condition, so I filled him in on my situation as we walked around the marina close to his apartment in Lasalle, a suburb of Montreal.

When we arrived back at his home, he said he had to finish developing some pictures in his darkroom for work the next day and offered to drive me back home when he was finished.

It was a beautiful day, so I went outside to sit down and wait for him. There happened to be a young mother sitting on the step of a walk-up apartment building next door. She was playing with her toddler, so I opened a conversation with her. I found out that she was in an abusive relationship and was afraid of her husband. After ten minutes or so, the little one was getting a bit cranky so we went inside where she put her down for a nap. We continued our conversation over a cup of tea at her kitchen table, and I was so caught up in her story that I completely forgot about Steve.

And no wonder with the drama that unfolded soon after.

Her husband worked at the airport as a baggage handler, and when he came in from work, he didn't hide the fact that he did not want me there. He sat down with a beer and glared at me across the table as if I were some kind of an intruder. I wasn't sure how to react, so I excused myself and started to get up to leave. He said a few angry words to his wife and she just looked down as if afraid to speak. When he asked her a question and she didn't reply, he became angry and without any warning reached over and struck her in the face with his fist.

"What are you doing?" I yelled.

"Call the police!" she cried as she staggered to the bathroom, her nose bleeding profusely.

I rushed to her side and tried to hold her up over the toilet.

"Don't you dare call the police!" he shouted as he stormed out the door. "I'll kill you!"

I was shaking as I dialed the number for the police. She asked if I would stay with her until the police arrived, but Steve had no idea what was going on or even where I was.

"I think I should let my friend know where I am," I said. "I'll come back when the police get here, okay?"

But when I stepped outside, her husband suddenly bolted out from between the two buildings and came at me in a rage.

"I'm going to kill you!"

I ran towards Steve's building just as the police were turning into their driveway. They caught those last moments when he ran around the side of their building.

"He just threatened me!" I said.

"Come with us," the officer said as he got out of his car and walked to the door with me.

Apparently, this was the first time police had been summoned to their apartment. After assessing the situation and asking questions, they wanted to know whether or not she would press charges against her husband. It puzzled me when she declined, but then I figured she must have been too afraid. Surprisingly, her baby slept through all of it.

After all that turmoil, I remembered I wanted to try that number I found in my purse, so I called again. This time someone answered, and it turned out to be a pivotal moment that miraculously changed everything for me that Sunday afternoon.

"Who am I speaking to?" I asked the person who answered.

"Who do you want to speak to?" came the reply.

"I have this telephone number but no name, so I'm wondering whose number this is."

"The only person here besides me is Bob, but he's not here right now," he said.

In a flash I remembered that name from the Cozy Club on Saint-Catherine Street where Dougie used to go with his friends. *It must be his number.*

"When will he be back?" I asked.

"No idea, sorry."

"Please don't hang up!" I said with desperation in my voice.

"Is something wrong?" he asked?

"I need to pick up my luggage but I don't have a car and I hoped Bob might help."

"Well, I have a van, will that do?" came the reply.

When I gave him the address he said, "I'm only minutes away from where you are. I can come over now if you'd like."

"You have no idea how much I appreciate this!" I said.

"No problem, what is your name?" he asked.

"Anna," I replied.

"Okay, see you soon," he said with a reassuring tone.

I hung up the phone and quickly tried to explain the turn of events to the young mother. She was afraid her husband might come back at any moment, so I placed a kitchen chair in front of the door, grabbed a kitchen knife and hid it under a cushion there on the chair. Then I went and sat on the arm of the sofa in front of the picture window anxiously awaiting the van. The moment I saw a van with a signal light flashing to turn into the driveway, I slid off the arm of the sofa, saying, "The van is here!" In doing so, I felt a tear in the back of my maternity skirt where the pleat was, but I paid no attention. As I stepped outside, he was already on the narrow sidewalk coming towards me. He was about six feet tall, average build.

"Hi! I'm Lee," he said with an outstretched hand. "You must be … Anne?"

He followed me upstairs to where the young mother was with her baby. When Lee came in, he stood at the door observing as I took the knife from under the cushion and put it back in the kitchen. His eyebrows raised when he saw the knife.

I asked, "Should I leave the chair here next to the door?"

"Yes, he's really mad at me!" she said.

"If you feel you're in danger you should call the police and don't be afraid to press charges," I said as I jotted down my address and handed it to Lee.

"Is this where we pick up the luggage?" he asked.

"Yes, it's where I work as a live-in domestic for an elderly couple."

I was preoccupied with our conversation as we pulled out of the driveway, so it completely slipped my mind to let Steve know where I was. At least I had my purse. When we arrived at the house, we collected the two suitcases and Lee put them into his van. He sat for a moment with an inquisitive look on his face. I was physically and emotionally exhausted by then. I didn't know whether to laugh or cry. I was extremely uncomfortable as well because the baby was more active than usual.

"Okay, where to now?" he asked, slowly pulling away from the curb.

"Um-m-m, well … I … I um, don't know."

He glanced at me as if he thought I was kidding, but then I saw it dawn on his face that I literally did not know where to go from there. We were both quiet as he continued to drive slowly around a few blocks as if thinking what to do next. He looked terribly concerned, and he suddenly pulled over and stopped.

"I'll be right back," he said, then disappeared.

I have been in paralyzing situations before, but this is absolutely unreal, I thought to myself. About fifteen minutes later he hopped back into the van and tossed a paper into my lap.

"Well, you have a place for the next six months," he said, and started the van.

"What's this?" I asked.

"It's a lease. So now we should buy a few groceries before the stores close. What do you think?"

I was stunned. I couldn't speak. It wasn't until we got to the mall that it sunk in. He put the large bag of groceries on the counter of the little kitchenette and told me I should take it easy and not to worry. I can't explain it, but I honestly had no fear or apprehension when I began to unpack my suitcases and set up my sleeping quarters. Lee left with the reassurance that he would come back the next day, so there I was, numb, as I reflected on the craziness of that day. It was as if I had been walking along the edge of a cliff when a hand suddenly reached out from nowhere, pulling me away from imminent danger.

I was still asleep the next day when I heard the knock on the door.

"It's Lee!" he said.

I jumped up and opened the door, greeting him as if he were an old friend.

"How was your night?" he asked.

"The baby was restless, which kept me awake for quite a while, but I did have a sound sleep eventually. I just woke up. What time is it anyway?" I asked.

"It's lunch time. I just came over from work to see how you are doing."

"You have no idea how much you have done for me, Lee. I will never forget your incredible generosity."

"I felt compelled to do something. You were obviously in a real bind and with no support, but it looks like it was the right thing to do. You seem to be in good spirits today. I will be getting back to work now, but I will drop by on my way home if you'd like."

"We have the groceries, so why don't I cook something for supper?" I asked.

"Sure, if you don't mind, that would be really nice," he replied. "Then I'll definitely come by after work tomorrow."

With the way things were unfolding, I felt a glimmer of confidence that the remaining weeks of my pregnancy would go well.

We had our first talk that evening after supper, and I learned quite a bit about him. He was fifteen years older than me. His parents had passed away, leaving him with one sibling, a sister, but she died a few years before. He had one distant relative whom he had not been in touch with for a number of years. So at the present time he was living with Bob, whose telephone number I found in my purse. What a crazy connection.

Grateful for Lee having paid for the six month lease that he took, I was also comforted when he came by every day to check on me to make sure I was okay during those last few weeks before my delivery.. And finally when I went into labour at the end of October 1966, he took me to the hospital where I gave birth to a healthy baby boy I named Steven. He also brought flowers for me and a box of chocolates for the nurse.

I found it extremely difficult to deal with the emotional side, when, after holding and feeding him for a few days, I sat down in a small private room to discuss the process of legal adoption. I felt deep remorse when signing those papers, and I was reminded of the pain of letting go of baby Lynn Marie, Elizabeth Anne and Andy.

It was now 1966, and when I returned to my hospital bed after signing the adoption papers, I prayed this baby would be placed in a good home where he would be loved and well taken care of. I gave thanks that Andy, Elizabeth Anne and Lynn Marie were in good hands back in New Waterford as well. Even though I missed them terribly, I began to understand how selfish it was for me to take any of them along when I decided to leave New Waterford. I realized I was not stable enough to deal with the problems I had to face when out there on my own.

As I lay there in the hospital bed, I was finally able to let go of the fantasy that one day I would be together with all of my children. I had to be honest and admit to myself that with the passing of time and the unforeseen events since Dougie and I had split up, this scenario I entertained in my mind was unlikely. I didn't know how to deal with the deep sadness that crept into my mind that night, so I asked the nurse if she would give me something to help me sleep, hoping tomorrow I would see things in a different light and find reason to go on.

Lee seemed to understand my struggle from the very beginning, so I really appreciated his positivity when he visited me the next day. Being somewhat of a joker, he often made me laugh with some off-the-cuff remark. He was my one and only support, and with all the unhealthy situations I'd found myself in before he appeared on the scene, I actually began to feel safe with him.

Chapter 13

I felt like I was living in some kind of limbo. I never wanted to go anywhere except with Lee for long drives out of the city every once in a while. I realized I really was not well when our next-door neighbour, a young man, approached me one day at our outdoor pool just to have a neighbourly chat. I immediately got up and went inside. My hands were trembling, and I asked myself why I was feeling this way. *Why am I unable to simply connect with anyone around me?* I began to realize that both Anita and I had deep-rooted problems stemming from childhood. Neither of us really knew how to have normal interactions with people, and we felt terribly lost when out there on our own.

It dawned on me that I had not contacted any family members since I found out I was pregnant with Andy's baby. It must have been the deep shame I felt that made me disconnect, and I figured I'd just have to get through those nine months on my own somehow.

I wondered how Anita was making out, so I decided to contact her. She had no way of knowing where I was or what had been happening with me over this past year. I was not surprised to hear how hard she struggled as a waitress at a well-known restaurant chain called Murray's. She was let go when she could not handle the stress. However, I was stunned when she revealed that she had recently given birth to a baby boy and had to give him up for adoption.

"Oh my God! This is unbelievable!" I said. "I just gave birth to a baby boy at the end of October, and he, too, is up for adoption!"

"So we were both pregnant at the same time again!" she exclaimed.

That was the first time we had some kind of dialogue where we actually shared our experiences. We realized that we were never really there for one another, especially when things got tough. We always seemed to go in opposite directions looking for solutions.

Not long after that conversation, Anita called back and asked if she could come over for a visit. When she arrived, she appeared to be quite tired and didn't look well at all. I was concerned.

"Are you okay?"

"Well, maybe that train ride wasn't such a good idea," she said, "because I started to have some pain in my abdomen on the way."

I knew right away it must be related to her recent cesarian section.

"Can you show me where it hurts?" I asked.

When I saw the long, ruptured scar with a couple of the sutures actually coming out, I was shocked! All along the stitches were painful looking red and blue bruises.

"No wonder you're in pain," I said. "You're going to have to see a doctor right away!"

It was too soon for her to travel; it was dangerous. She told me that when the doctor examined her, he said he couldn't believe she had made that five-hour train ride from Toronto to Montreal after having major surgery. Obviously, she had to take time to heal, not only physically but mentally—I could see that. So she rented a tiny apartment nearby where we were able to keep an eye on her for the next few months until she had recuperated.

In the meantime, I discovered we did not have that ideal relationship people assume twins have. A subconscious pattern must have developed at an early age where she had become more dominant. Or so I thought until one day when she dropped in unannounced. Lee was at work and I had just finished vacuuming the floors. It was a cold winter's day but the sun was shining brightly.

"It's nice outside, let's go out for a walk," she said.

"No Anita. I don't feel like going out."

Usually I would go along even if I didn't feel like it. However, that day I was just too tired and didn't want to go. I was rather disappointed when she began to pester me, because I thought she understood from our last conversation over the phone that we were to be more considerate of each other's feelings.

"But I really do not want to go," I said.

When she insisted again, I firmly said, "No!"

"Well, okay then! I'm going to call Dougie and tell him that you are living with Lee!"

It hit me like a ton of bricks. I was being manipulated! I felt so hurt, and my mind went into a spin. I looked around for anything I could get my hands on and spotted a pair of high heeled shoes on the floor near the door. I grabbed one in a blind fury and swung at her. She ducked and then ran around the kitchen table and out the door.

I had never reacted physically and with such anger. Neither of us were the loud or the aggressive type growing up, so we never had any altercations. I figured it must have been the accumulation of incidents over the years where she refused to take my feelings into account that caused the outburst. We were disconnected again for quite some time after that.

Living with Lee helped me be calm and let go of all the drama in my life. Neither of us talked about our past, which was good for me at least, since it would have opened up psychic wounds. Since I didn't see any problems in our relationship, I wanted to keep it that way.

*

Two years had passed since Anita and I had that terrible incident, so I was glad to hear from her when she finally called. She had just come back from out west where she said she had been working as a graphic artist's assistant while living with our older brother Junior (a soldier) and his family. She was back in Toronto and asked if she could come over and stay with us for a while. I said it would be okay but she had to be careful not to cause any trouble this time. We agreed to put the past behind us and make an effort to get along.

Around that time I had generated enough courage to board a plane and fly back to Cape Breton in the hopes that I could see Andy, Elizabeth Anne and Lynn Marie. I shouldn't have been surprised, though, when Dougie denied me access because he was still mad at me for not going back to live in New Waterford when he took Lynn home.

As I wasn't able to go to Dougie's house, I went to the kids' school instead, where I met with the principal. She showed kindness and understanding, and she actually took both Elizabeth Anne and Lynn Marie out of class to be with me there in her office. I did not get a chance to see Andy because he was absent that day.

Back in Montreal, Lee was understanding and supportive. I still was not able to socialize in any way, and I reverted back to isolation for a few months. I did not want to go out at all, not even for one of our occasional long drives. There was an emptiness that is hard to describe when I was living without the children. As I said, I do not ever remember talking to Lee about my past. Because he was such an upbeat sort of person, I think it must have helped me to ignore the painful memories and to begin thinking more of the future and less about the past.

By now we were into July of 1968. Anita happened to be with me one day when I was sewing on the portable machine that Lee had bought for me. I tried to keep my mind busy by making my own dresses from the Simplicity Patterns you could buy at that time. We didn't have much to say, just keeping each other company, when Lee popped in unexpectedly with his cheerful hello.

"I feel like taking a break today," he said, "so what do you say we go for a drive up into the mountains? You can come along, too, Anita, if you'd like!"

She was quite happy about that, so I thought it would do us all good if we were to get out of the city for a while. The beauty of the countryside put me into a mood of serenity, with thoughts of gratitude taking over as we left the city behind. About an hour and a half into our drive, Lee turned onto a gravel road where there was a farm here and there along the way. He slowed down and turned into a driveway. I assumed he was about to turn around to head back to Montreal, but he continued on into the yard and pulled up in front of a farmhouse.

"Do you know the people here?" I asked, totally surprised.

"Yes, let's see if they're home. I'll tell you about it later, okay?"

He knocked, then opened the door.

"Anybody home?"

No answer.

"They must be out in the field," he said as he got back into the car. "I'll honk the horn and maybe they'll hear. Do you remember me telling you I have a relative I haven't seen in many years?"

"Yes, I do."

"Well, he had a little cabin up in the back of this property when I last saw him, which was about twenty years ago, and I'm wondering if he's still around."

"But who lives here on the farm?" I asked.

"Two brothers who came over from England many years ago; they cleared the land and built this farm together. Both of them are bachelors, never married. Their names are Malcom and Jim. Lately I've been wondering just how they're doing. I'm sure they'll be very surprised by our visit."

A few minutes later, I spotted someone walking towards the house.

"Oh? Someone is coming; it must be one of the farmers," I said.

"Yes, it looks like Malcom, the older one," said Lee as he got out of the car.

They greeted each other with a friendly pat on the back and shook hands with an air of excitement.

"Jim will be here soon; he has to bring the horses over to the barn first," said Malcom.

After our introductions we went into the house where Malcom made hot drinks for us. Then he sat down at the kitchen table and began rolling his own cigarettes while reminiscing. A cheerful greeting ensued when Jim entered, and they continued their conversation for quite some time. It was dark by the time the three of us headed back to Montreal.

Once I had accepted the fact that Andy, Elizabeth Anne and Lynn Marie could not be part of my life, I began to think seriously about the possibility of having another child. Lee and I had been together almost three years by now, and I thought he would be taken aback by my suggestion, but he simply responded with, "Whatever you want is okay with me." It was as if he had given it some thought already.

I had never experienced actually trying to conceive before, so when I stopped taking the birth control pills in August, I waited anxiously for September to arrive thinking I would be pregnant. My past experiences made me think it was easy for me to conceive, so when it didn't happen, I shed a few tears of disappointment.

Then when October came I shed a couple of tears again, but this time it was because I was overjoyed to find out that I was as fertile as ever. At the age of twenty-seven in that last week of October 1969, hope was clearly on the horizon and I began to look to the future with confidence for a change.

To celebrate my pregnancy, I was open to going to a party with Lee. Something I had never done before. He had a few friends I'd never met, so I thought maybe it was time for me to come out of my shell and get to know them—or at least make an effort to meet with them. Lee was pleasantly surprised by my suggestion.

Shortly afterwards he took me along to his friend's house where maybe ten people or more had gathered. I was feeling a bit insecure as we entered the house. My first impression was how low-key the atmosphere was. Soft music played in the background as people stood around chatting, drinks in hand. I had expected more upbeat music along with some dancing, but I quickly adjusted.

Someone greeted us, took our coats and invited us to join the group. I followed Lee as he introduced me to a couple of his friends. I'm trying to remember how things progressed from there but am having trouble because the images are so fragmented. I see another room to my right where it looked like a few people were sitting and watching a movie. On second glance I realized it was actually a projector with a film running, and the images flashing on the screen threw me for a loop.

"What in the world?"

I was instantly repelled at the sight of a large dog having sex with a human.

I turned to Lee, dumbfounded, and said, "Why would you bring me here? I'm not interested in this garbage!"

"We won't stay if you're offended," he said.

"This is disgusting, let's go!" I demanded as I turned to leave.

I was bewildered when Lee appeared to be apologizing to the host for my refusal to stay. We left that house but didn't go home. I see us entering a bar, I guess you'd call it, where Lee introduced me to another friend of his. We were sitting at the little table a few minutes when Lee said he had to use the washroom. Because I was jolted by what had just happened, I was in no mood for any kind of conversation with his friend. I was bewildered and I just sat there in silence waiting for Lee to return. I soon became restless when he seemed to be taking so long.

"I'll go see what's taking so long," his friend said.

A minute later, he came back and said, "He's not there—I don't know where he is."

"What? You must be kidding!" I said, losing my composure.

"Don't worry, I will drive you home."

At first, I was baffled by Lee's sudden disappearance, but now I was really getting upset.

"What is going on here?" I insisted.

There was no response as he calmly led me to his car. While driving the short distance home, I was shocked when he slowly placed his hand on my knee without saying a word. I shoved his hand away in utter disgust. I was getting a little nervous but with firmness in my voice I ordered, "Drop me off at Lee's. I've had enough of this crap."

He was clearly unperturbed by my response and continued driving. My mind was racing—I didn't know what to do—so I just sat there feeling helpless. When we stopped in front of our apartment building, I grabbed my purse, desperately searching for my keys so I'd get to the door before him.

"Thanks for the lift" I said sarcastically, as I grabbed my purse- hopped out of the car and gave the door a slam. As I rushed towards the entrance to our apartment building, I was surprised when I turned, and saw that he was now following behind! But thankfully I reached the door before he caught up, just in time to lock him out! Safe inside I let out a huge sigh of relief. Then my mind immediately turned to Lee, and the huge disappointment that day turned out to be. It was supposed to have been a celebratory day for us! Having been misled into thinking it was going to be a normal social gathering was very disturbing indeed; even in that type of a situation it would have been difficult for me.

Aside from that terrible incident, which showed me just how naïve I was, I actually thought we got along very well. He was an easy person to live with, and I don't recall having any problems until that night. Now my concern was whether I could pass this evening off as insignificant and continue as if nothing happened or if it would cause friction between us.

I was asleep when he returned, but I could feel the tension in the air the next day. He tried to have a sense of humour about it when I brought it up, and it was as if he didn't quite get how it affected me on the mental and emotional levels. Seeing how we were both on a different page about it, I just went silent; I knew there was no use pushing it. I couldn't get close to him after that, and I even avoided our usual small talk at the table.

Life became a riddle once again, and I didn't know what to expect down the road. That uncertainty caused me to slide back into my old pattern where I simply disconnected from everyone, including Lee. He seemed to be just fine, though, going about his day as usual and not realizing (or ignoring) that we may have a problem.

I wanted our relationship to be normal again after that disappointing night, but as much as I tried, I was not able to let go of the negative feelings I had about it. I did not know where he went or why he left me with his friend there that night. And when questioned, he was able to skirt around the issue with his usual sense of humour that made light of the situation.

One day, Lee suggested we go back to the farm to visit Malcom and Jim. He said it seemed to help me open up a bit, to come out of my shell so to speak. As expected, Anita wanted to come too. I couldn't say no as she was alone and I honestly felt sorry for her. When I mentioned it to Lee, he agreed as I figured he would, because of the friendly outgoing person he was.

When we arrived, there was another vehicle parked in front of the house.

"They must have some company," said Lee. "I'm sure they won't mind because everybody is friendly up here."

We were introduced to their lifelong friend Bruce, who lived with his elderly parents on the highway just minutes away. Around my age, he was of average height and build with a quiet, unassuming personality. More of an observer I would say.

That afternoon turned out to be another milestone for me. There was an instant connection between Bruce and I which caught me by surprise. Words were not necessary to convey the message that he obviously found me interesting and liked me in a rather innocent way. He was quite comfortable just listening and watching closely as Lee, Malcom, Jim, Anita and myself spent that Sunday afternoon sharing stories and laughter until it became dark outside. It was great just to be able to get out and be with such nice, friendly people for a change. I was happy for Anita, too, because she had been struggling for so long and she wanted this too.

Before we left that day, we learned that Bruce's father was in the hospital in Montreal with cancer and that Bruce had been going to see him on a regular basis. Lee and I invited him to stop in whenever he happened to be in the Montreal area, which was an hour and a half drive away. Apparently his father was not doing well, so Bruce had been going to see him more often lately.

The following week, Bruce called during the afternoon saying he was at the hospital. I asked if he had time to stop by for a visit, which he took me up on. When he was leaving after a short stay, I suggested he come back the next time he visited with his father.

"But what will Lee say?" he asked.

I was immediately drawn to this side of him. He clearly was not on the prowl, so to speak, and he demonstrated a certain kind of respect that I liked very much. I have to admit that it was the moment when I became—how should I put it?—smitten? In a roundabout way, I let him know that Lee and I had no future and it was only a matter of time before it would end. Perhaps I was a little forward because he looked as if he didn't know what to say, so I backed off. But I honestly felt right then and there that fate had stepped in and change was about to take place. That this unexpected connection was meant to be.

In hindsight it is obvious (to me at least) that I was always being taken care of by a higher power. This timing of Bruce being in Montreal just as Lee and I were drifting apart showed me where things were headed. I knew intuitively that Bruce and I would eventually be together. Of course, he was not aware of this yet.

As he was about to go out the door, I wanted to show him how I felt, I guess, and I spontaneously gave him a little peck on the cheek. He smiled with a slight tinge of embarrassment as he turned to leave.

"Hope to see you again soon!" I added with an optimistic tone.

How would I handle this unfinished business between Lee and me? I knew Lee was trying in his own way to keep things afloat and hoping I would simply forget that night at the party and the bar. But he didn't realize the impact it had on me; it meant I was no longer interested in intimacy of any kind with him. He seemed to think it was just a glitch in our relationship and that I would soon get over it even though I steadfastly refused to reconnect with him physically.

The next time Bruce came into Montreal, Lee happened to be at home, and I must say I did like the friendly interaction between them. Lee was the more talkative one while Bruce was more of a listener. I found the visit to be quite amicable for the three of us, so I was able to relax and simply be in the moment.

Bruce told us that Malcom and Jim would be cooking their upcoming Christmas dinner as they always did and we were all welcome to eat with them at the farm. We were only too happy to accept the invitation of course, but we were rather curious when he added, "Jim said to make sure to bring Anita with you." When I thought about it later, I did notice they paid a lot of attention to each other the last time we were there in the fall, but I didn't suspect she'd be interested in him because of their age difference. He was actually twenty years older than her. But then we noted that Lee was fifteen years older than me and concluded with a sense of humour that we must be attracted to the fatherly type. Lee and I were delighted with the invitation and made plans for all of us to spend Christmas Day at the farm.

The twenty-fifth turned out to be a gorgeous sunny day. The scenery was absolutely beautiful, and breathing in that fresh country air as we stepped out of the car was incredibly invigorating. It felt like a winter wonderland. A skidoo was parked in front of the door, so we figured it must belong to Bruce. Jim and Malcom greeted us with Bruce right there behind. It was obvious I was excited to see him again and vise versa.

Everyone seemed to be in the holiday spirit. I was immediately struck by the warmth from the old-fashioned wood stove in the kitchen which carried that wonderful scent of wood through the living room and upstairs into the bedrooms. Overall the house was rather small, nothing fancy, but it was clean and so cozy! This was the first time Anita and I had ever celebrated Christmas on a farm, and we were thrilled to be there. Malcom and Jim were busy preparing the turkey with all the trimmings, and we brought the deserts as well as a few presents, nothing extravagant. I truly enjoyed the simplicity of it all.

I was not showing I was pregnant, and I did not want to reveal my secret just yet. Just before we sat down to dinner, Bruce asked if I would go for a ride with him on his skidoo, and I didn't know how to respond because of my condition. When Jim heard me say I had never been on a skidoo before and wasn't sure I should go, he said, "What? Never been on a skidoo, Annie? (he always called me Annie) Go ahead, you should try it!"

"Well okay, let's go!" I said with a sudden spark of enthusiasm.

Along the trail that led to the back of their sixty acre farm, the freshly fallen snow was thick on the branches of the evergreen trees all along the way. Like a picture postcard, the beauty was simply stunning. Coming near the end of the trail, he slowed down to go up a slight embankment and turn around, but the skidoo started to lean to the left side causing it to tip slightly.

"Hang on!" Bruce shouted. "Just put your left foot on the ground for a second until I turn around!"

"Oh no! I'm afraid I'm about to fall off!" I shouted over the high-pitched rumble of the motor. Then the words "Please be careful—I'm pregnant!" slipped out of my mouth.

The skidoo suddenly came to an abrupt halt. He removed his helmet, turned around with a dazed look and said, "WHAT? What did you say?"

"Oh nothing, just please be careful!"

He put his helmet back on and we continued along the trail with the sound of the motor buzzing in my ears. I didn't know whether he actually heard what I had said, but we returned safe and sound just in time for dinner.

Anita had been helping set the table while Lee was entertaining Jim and Malcom with his ever-present sense of humour people liked so much. I was truly amazed when Malcom and Jim served us a wonderful meal that day. I must have been holding on to the old stereotype image of a man not being able to cook. Or maybe because none of my partners had ever shown interest in cooking or helping in the kitchen, I was surprised that they could put such a meal together. Anyway, because of Jim and Malcom's example, I did let go of that gender nonsense right then and there.

It was quite interesting indeed how things unfolded around the table that day. Bruce stared at me with questions written on his face, which made me think he must have heard me. This definitely was not the scenario

I had in mind. I intended to share this with him when we had a quiet moment together. Instead, I was thinking I had better let everyone know immediately. Hopefully my news would add to the festive atmosphere and give us more cause to celebrate.

Nearing the end of our meal, I found myself glancing around while searching for the right words to say. I locked eyes with Bruce hoping he would not be disappointed with me for not letting him know sooner. Finally I was ready.

"There is something I have been wanting to tell you, so I don't think I should put it off any longer," I said. "And that is, I have been pregnant since October and am expecting to have a baby sometime in June."

Everyone sat and stared at me as if they didn't know what to say.

"I was wondering if you were going to mention it," said Lee.

"I think this is a good time, don't you? Since we all happen to be here together?" I said.

After congratulations from Jim and Bruce, the defining moment came when Anita unexpectedly jumped in with a bombshell of her own.

"I, too, am expecting a baby in July."

I wish I had a camera to capture the reaction on their faces in that moment.

"What?" Lee said, bursting into laughter. "You're kidding!"

Malcom frowned and rolled his eyes as if he disapproved. Jim looked embarrassed, while Bruce sat there staring into space as if trying to process what was taking place. I was stunned because of the time factor—Anita and I were pregnant at the same time for the third time!

I noted that Anita and Jim had been going for long walks when the leaves were changing colours in the fall. But none of us ever suspected that they had become romantically involved. It was truly incredible.

Looking back I find it rather strange and wonder why Anita and I had never shared news of our pregnancies with each other immediately as most families would. Also, as I look back now, there seems to be a pattern where she consciously or unconsciously—I'm not sure—eventually found me and more or less inserted herself into whatever situation I happened to be in at the time. It appeared to be happening with this new farm situation. But then I knew only too well what it was like to struggle alone and feel lost in this world, so deep down I was glad she had connected with Jim; he really was a decent guy.

Malcom was not at all pleased with this new state of affairs. But he more or less just grumbled a bit and that was the extent of it. By the time we left the farm that night, it appeared as if everyone had digested—mentally at least—the unexpected news that had been revealed there at the table on that Christmas Day of 1969.

Chapter 14

As I had expected, Anita moved up to the farm to be with Jim, which Malcom wasn't happy about at all. They managed to work things out over the winter, including coming up with a plan to build a little bungalow next to the farmhouse in the spring.

Lee and I stayed together for another few months, but more as friends since we were no longer involved in a physical relationship. When I told Lee that I really wanted to be with Bruce, he wasn't surprised. Actually, he was matter of fact about it.

"I didn't think you would stay with me forever, dear," he said in an understanding tone which helped immensely.

Once Lee and I were able to get past the awkward stage of sorting out our relationship, I wanted to spend more time with Bruce. His father passed away during the winter, but now his mother had been diagnosed with bone cancer and in a Montreal hospital, so I knew he was having a difficult time.

As before, he would come over to visit with me after seeing her in the hospital. His mother's illness did not drag on as long as his father's. She was diagnosed and sent to the hospital fairly quickly, and on Bruce's last visit with her, he said she told him, "Only a miracle will save me now." It turned out she was only in the hospital for a few weeks before she passed away. Losing both parents so close together must have been hard on Bruce, but he never showed any sign of grief when we were together. He was not the type of person to display emotion.

I never met his parents. In the beginning of our relationship I wondered why, since we always passed by their house on the highway when we drove up to the farm. Later on, I figured it was probably because they could not accept the fact that Robert was not Bruce's biological father; back in those days, this kind of judgment was quite common, so I can't say I was surprised that it had turned out the way it did.

With the melting of the snow in early spring, Jim was able to get started on the foundation of their little bungalow. Of course, he and his brother still had their normal everyday workload to tend to, and this kept them busy right up until the cold weather returned in the late fall.

Meantime I went into labour on the June 27, giving birth to a 7 lb., 14 oz. boy, whom I named Robert. Just ten days later, Anita gave birth to a baby girl she named Janice. Both babies were healthy, and we were thankful that everything seemed to be moving in the right direction in terms of our relationships. We were creating the safe and stable environment we had both longed for.

Lee brought me home from the hospital with Robert, and when we arrived it was heart-warming to find Bruce waiting for us with plenty of food that he had ordered as a surprise. What a wonderful welcome that was; I was thankful for the loving support that day.

When Bruce and I finally got together, it happened to be on a Labour Day weekend. Robert was just eight weeks old at the time. I find it quite remarkable that most major changes took place in my life on Labour Day weekend, as if it was written in the stars somehow. Anyway, with what I assumed had been Lee's blessing for me to move on, I was mystified when, on the day I was preparing to leave, he came into the kitchen with a rather sombre expression and sat down, as if wanting to talk. Bruce was there too.

"So you're really going through with it … you're leaving?" Lee asked.

I was a little confused since I had concluded from our conversations in the past few weeks that this would be the outcome.

"But I understood you had accepted the fact that I would be leaving with Robert, and that you wished me well, Lee," I said.

Bruce was also baffled since Lee hadn't appeared to have a problem up until now. The three of us sat there not knowing what to say next.

"I think you should stay," Lee finally said.

It was a sticky situation for sure. Since he'd always had a tendency to make light of serious situations, I had no indication Lee would become obstinate like this.

"Where are you taking them?" Lee asked Bruce with a stern look.

"I rented a basement apartment in a new house my friend built across the street from where I work. It's on the main street in Saint-Félix-de-Valois near Malcom and Jim's farm."

It seemed Lee was challenging Bruce, but he just went silent and wore a look of sheer determination. I didn't like the negative energy between them when Lee became persistent, and I could see that Bruce was not about to back down. Frankly, I was getting a little nervous and had a strong urge to step in, so I stood up and said, "This has turned out to be a very awkward situation, so maybe I should just stay here for tonight."

Bruce sat there speechless with such a look of disappointment that I almost changed my mind. But I knew I had to intervene somehow, as the atmosphere was becoming too tense. I can still see Bruce's expression as he turned and walked out the door in disbelief. He did not realize I only said I was going to stay in order to prevent further conflict between them. Although it worked, I felt incredibly guilty for disappointing Bruce.

That unexpected turn of events left things up in the air for all of us.

Although I was anxious to let him know the truth of the matter, I was not able to contact Bruce until the next day. It was inconceivable to me that he would actually turn away at this point, but at the same time I had to be prepared for whatever happened. I was cautiously optimistic when I had a chance to call him the next day while Lee was in the bathroom. Thankfully Bruce answered, and I quickly asked point blank, "Do you still want to be with me?"

"Yes, I still want us to be together," he said.

My heart instantly felt reassured, and I went on with my day with high hopes of us being together soon.

The next day, Lee decided we should go out for a drive. We ended up walking along a beach in Oka just outside of Montreal with Robert in his carriage. I was praying the whole time that Lee would come to accept that what I really wanted was to be with Bruce. Because Lee had not become attached to Robert (as Dougie was with Andy), I believe it was easier to take him with me. I was grateful there was no conflict over this at least.

I told him I would never forget the way he came to my rescue on that day we met and how much I truly appreciated his support. But, I told him, I lost trust in him and ended up distancing myself emotionally. I said I honestly had no desire to remain in that relationship any longer because I was fortunate enough to have connected with someone whom I believed I could have a future with.

Lee finally seemed to accept that our relationship was not about to go back to the way it was, and that my destiny, if you will, was with Bruce. I also stressed the point that he should be in Robert's life as much as possible. Bruce and I both realized how important that would be, so I reassured Lee that we would definitely co-operate as far as parenting was concerned. We ended the discussion with Lee telling me he would never give me any problems regarding Robert and that he would come by and see how we were doing every once in a while.

That long and fruitful conversation gave me enough incentive to put my plans for the future into motion.

The apartment Bruce found was in a newly built home of a French speaking family. I connected with them immediately even though my French was limited. They were courteous, kind, and they made us feel very much at home. We had the entire basement floor of their new home, and Bruce was quite satisfied because he just had to cross the street to get to his job as hatchery manager.

Not long after we were settled in, I bent down to pick up Robert from the floor in the kitchen when I suddenly felt a sharp pain in the middle of my back and couldn't straighten up at all.

"I can't move!" I called out to Bruce, who was in the living room.

He was there within seconds, but the pain kept me doubled over as I made my way to the couch. He left Robert with the landlord's wife and we raced to the emergency department at the hospital. The doctor said the X-rays showed my muscles were in knots, and he gave me pills for pain and to help me relax. We did not get to the cause of the pain itself, and as a matter of fact I did find the root cause until a few years later.

We hadn't seen Lee in awhile, so Bruce and I were genuinely happy to see him the next day when he popped in unexpectedly. With Robert as the centre of attention, Lee and Bruce seemed comfortable enough in each other's company, which made me feel good. I was lying on the couch, mostly just listening to their conversation because I was feeling so drowsy from the pills I had taken before Lee arrived. Upon leaving, Lee was his usual cheerful self, saying he would make a point of stopping by again soon.

*

By the time Robert turned two years old, I started to think it would be nice if he had a little brother or sister to grow up with. I decided to bring this up to Bruce even though he had mentioned that he didn't think he would ever get married or have children.

"What do you think about giving Robert a little brother or sister?" I asked with a hint of hope in my voice.

He looked at me totally surprised and said, "You mean you would go through all that again?"

"Well, yes, because it's not only for Robert, but also because you never had any children of your own," I said.

He was genuinely moved by this thought-provoking idea, so I thought I'd let it go at that.

"Sure—I would like that too," he said, seemingly captivated because I was not at all deterred.

I knew deep down that he was truly delighted at the thought of having a child, even though it had never been something he outwardly expressed. I always found him to be a selfless person with a desire to please, so I was motivated by his positive response.

On July 5, 1972, I went into labour for the sixth and final time. The hospital in Joliette was a fifteen-minute drive away, and we arrived just as the contractions intensified. Even though I had bought cassettes to learn French, I still had lots of trouble understanding the language, let alone speaking it. However, having always lived in the French speaking area, Bruce was bilingual, so I made sure he was right there by my side to translate.

After the preliminaries were taken care of, a young nurse took me to my room and for some reason Bruce did not or could not follow. As the nurse was getting me ready, she asked me something I could not understand. Although I was a little shy about speaking French, I did my best to communicate. None the less, I picked up on a negative vibe from her. She was becoming impatient with me, which was an indication that I was not about to receive the care I needed. I began to tense up and wondered where Bruce was.

Seconds after she left the room, I had a strong contraction. I was about to deliver, so I called out for someone to come help, but no one came.

"Where's the nurse? Someone has to be here with me!" I pleaded.

The labour pains suddenly became unbearable. I couldn't remember the French words for help, so I called out in English "PLEASE HELP ME!" A few seconds later, the nurse came back and lifted the sheet to check.

"Ça arrive!" she shouted.

Another nurse rushed into the room and they lifted me onto another bed at the very moment I was having the most painful contraction ever! As they quickly wheeled me from one room to another, I felt the jab of a needle in my right hip. The next thing I remember was staring up at a big round light above me while letting out a long, hellish scream as the baby was coming. I wasn't even in a proper position! It was the most excruciating pain I had ever experienced. I felt as if I was about to leave my body—I'm not exaggerating.

I do not know when Bruce entered the room, I was totally unaware, but he said he thought he was going to pass out. He was overwhelmed by the whole experience, which was definitely not what one would expect to have in any hospital, anywhere!

Seconds after the delivery, my mind quickly focused on our newborn. I was thankful again that this baby, a boy whom we named Stephen, was just fine. However, I couldn't wait to leave the hospital and put that awful experience behind me.

It was such a relief to be safe at home again and to see how Robert was overjoyed with his new baby brother. One of Bruce's co-workers commented on how he was absolutely thrilled to be a father for the first time, and it was very gratifying to hear.

We did just fine for the next few years until my need to communicate with Bruce on a deeper level became an issue. I began to feel ignored whenever

I'd try to reach out to connect. I simply wanted him to pay attention to me when I had to express whatever was on my mind. He didn't seem to comprehend this, and the more I was ignored, the more it became an issue. I started to think that maybe it would be less painful if I were by myself or if I lived with complete strangers where there would be no attachment and I wouldn't be reaching out to connect emotionally all the time.

Robert was about five and Stephen was three when this crazy idea suddenly popped into my head. Have you ever done something where you didn't realize just how stupid it was until later? Like, *What in the world was I thinking?* Looking back, I swear only half of my brain must have been working while the other half was dozing off the day I placed an ad in the *Halifax Herald* newspaper.

I had decided to take Robert and Stephen with me to Nova Scotia to find work as a live-in domestic. I thought I'd be able live in a home where I could work while keeping Robert and Stephen with me. Maybe I was trying to find a place as I did when I had Liz with me in Montreal years ago? I don't know.

I received only one reply to the ad, which I answered. I got out of the taxi I had taken from the airport in front of this little red brick house that had a couple of tractors in the yard. I didn't know what to think. Robert and Stephen seemed interested, and they climbed up onto them as the owner, an elderly looking man, came to meet us. When I stepped inside and saw the mess that was waiting just for me, I realized what a terrible mistake I'd made!

I didn't want to show that I just wanted to turn around and leave, so I found myself being rather polite. I sat down to hear exactly what was expected of me, but within a few days we were right back on a flight for home!

As crazy as that was, I did the same thing again only weeks later when I flew to the west coast. Robert, Stephen and I arrived in Vancouver, where I had gotten a response to an ad I placed in the *Vancouver Sun* newspaper. It, too, turned out to be another stupid situation I had put us in, so I was soon on my way back home again. Those trips from east to west were a total waste of time and money, but no one could have convinced me at the time how far fetched my ideas were. Whenever I had an idea, I jumped on it, and I only learned just how insane those decisions were through trial and error. I must say Bruce was like no other in putting up with my illogical thinking and behaviour at times, and I will always hold a special place for him in my heart for that.

Luckily, we were back in time to enroll Robert in the nearby English school in Joliette. We had been living in the basement apartment for a few years when Bruce decided we should build a house of our own close by. It was a big undertaking since he didn't hire anyone, and we started from scratch once he bought the two lots and cleared the trees. It was a new section that was being opened up about a mile off the highway, up in the hills. He said his friend had already bought one of the lots, which was next to an artificial lake.

Malcom and Jim's farm was only five minutes away, so Anita and I saw each other quite often. She would bring Janice over to the lake and I'd take Robert to visit them in their little bungalow that Jim had built next to the farmhouse.

When Bruce came in from work, we'd have supper and then head up to work on our house with Robert and Stephen in tow. We started around May of 1975 and were finally able to move in by May 1977.

The chronic pain in my back gradually worsened, and the pain killers I took soon became a problem because I started reaching for them not only for the physical pain. Emotional pain had been brewing for some time whenever I felt disconnected.

Bruce and I didn't go out very often, but when we did, our neighbour Myriam babysat for us. She was about eighteen years old and lived with her mother who worked in the hatchery with Bruce. She and her mother were completely bilingual, so I had no problem communicating with them.

Myriam had mentioned that she was going out with this guy who wanted to get married but her mother did not approve of him. She confided that she was having second thoughts about getting married but he persuaded her to reconsider. She did, and they went ahead and got married not long after that. She loved spending time with Robert and Stephen.

I will never forget the day Bruce came home from the hatchery at lunchtime with an expression on his face as if he had just seen a ghost.

"I just got some bad news," he said with a serious tone.

"Oh no, what happened?" I asked, almost afraid to hear what he had to say.

"I just had a call from Myriam's mother telling me why she didn't come into work this morning," he said as he sat down at the table. "I can't believe it … I can't believe it!"

"Believe WHAT?" I asked.

"Something terrible has happened," he said. "Myriam is no longer with us. Her mother just told me that she was shot and killed while sleeping in her bed last night."

"Oh … my … God …," I almost chocked on the words.

"Apparently her husband was out drinking on the weekend and came home late; Myriam was in bed asleep when he took a pillow, put it over her head and shot her dead."

We were horrified and shocked beyond belief. We often hear horror stories on the news regarding tragedies such as this, but when it is someone you know and love, the mind cannot accept the fact that it actually happened.

Her mother, of course, was mortified to get the devastating news. At the wake when we offered our condolences, her mother clasped her hands around mine and said, "I want to tell you that Myriam thought the world of you. She spoke of you often, saying how much she liked going over to your place to babysit. She showed me that long black hair piece you gave her, and she even went out to buy the same bedspread as you have on your bed, except it's a different colour."

It meant a lot that she expressed this sentiment, but it was heart-wrenching to see her go through such agony. When I passed in front of Myriam's casket, it was rather unnerving because you could see how one side of her face was slightly distorted from the impact of the bullet. Rumour had it that Myriam had decided to ask for a divorce because he treated her badly and that she had become terribly afraid of him. Apparently, he was out at a bar drinking and was getting angrier as the night went on. Just before he left, he mentioned to someone that he definitely was not going to give her the divorce she wanted.

Instead, he turned his anger on her that awful night. He was quickly taken into custody and charged with her murder. To add to this unthinkable tragedy, it was only months later when Myriam's mother was suddenly stricken with a fatal heart attack. People said she died from a broken heart.

That awful tragedy made me think more seriously about our journey through this life. I took more time for contemplation and to think about our relationships and just what matters most in the time we have left here on this earth.

I will inject something here relating to what I call "the pill problem." When Bruce and I came home from working on the house and the kids were tucked in for the night, this feeling of disconnect from our lack of communication really began to bother me. I became more insistent on having a little conversation just before bedtime to the point of becoming a bit of pest at times. I cannot recall ever feeling this way when I was with any other partners.

Bruce liked to play tennis with the company vet, was captain of his bowling team and had been a pitcher on his baseball team before we met. These activities were put on hold when we started building our house, and, of course, by the end of the day he simply sat in front of the TV to relax.

I wanted that for him, too, but I also needed a few minutes of some kind of connection before we turned in for the night; he didn't seem to notice. For instance, whenever I'd say, "Can we talk?" he'd say okay, but he was more interested in the sports on TV. it made me think I didn't matter. This was especially so when he'd say, "If you want to talk, why don't you go over and talk to Bobby?" (the wife of Bruce's best friend). I had spoken with her, but it did not satisfy my ever-increasing need to be heard.

It was as if the traumas of the past had been neatly tucked away during those four years with Lee and they were now simmering just beneath the surface. Bruce had no knowledge about my past or what I needed for the present and future. It would have been therapeutic just to have his ear, but when that didn't happen, I'd simply take more pills to dull the emotional pain of disconnect.

One evening when I saw he was about to settle down to watch a baseball game, I was unable to ignore this nagging need to communicate any longer. So at the risk of feeling rejected once again, I decided to give a hint one more time before the game started. When that didn't work, I asked in a serious, heartfelt way that if I needed him to take a few minutes to talk with me—that I needed his attention. I was not ready to hear, "Go and talk to Bobby," again, but that's exactly what happened. As usual, it "triggered" a deep-seated feeling of rejection, and I found myself reacting out of hurt, then anger.

I stood up and quietly walked into the kitchen with the intention of taking a couple of pills to calm down. I usually did this when upset. But without any warning, as I opened the cupboard door to reach for the pills my mind seemed to just explode with emotion. Completely devoid of any rational thought, I just popped the cap off the container, grabbed a glass of water and swallowed pills until the bottle was empty. The irony was that I did not recognize in that moment that I had done anything wrong! I threw the empty container into the garbage and stomped off to the bedroom as if I had solved that problem once and for all!

I laid there determined to say no more and just wait for the pills to take effect. About five minutes had passed when the door slowly opened and Bruce peeked in.

"Are you okay?" he asked, totally unaware I was on the brink of losing unconscious.

"As if you care!" I shot back. "Just leave me alone!"

Mumbling something under his breath, he closed the door. A minute or so later, I found myself sitting upright and wanting to respond. Even though the room was almost in darkness, I was able to see in front of me, so I tried to stand up. When I did, the room instantly switched from horizontal to vertical! That's when what I'd done hit me like a sledgehammer.

I edged towards the door at a snail's pace with my hands outstretched to balance myself. With what felt like my last ounce of energy I tried to let Bruce know what was happening, but I suddenly felt this rhythmic squishing deep inside my chest.

Can I get the words out in time?

I was losing consciousness as I stumbled into the living room, flopped on the couch, grabbed Bruce's arm and managed to say, "I swallowed a bottle of pills."

"You WHAT? THAT'S STUPID!"

He dragged me towards the kitchen.

"Drink some milk right away! WHERE'S YOUR MEDICARE CARD!" he shouted, rummaging through my purse.

I was not able to speak. He guided me into the bathroom where I forced myself to throw up after gulping down some milk he'd handed to me. Within minutes, we were outside getting into the car. Everything had slowed down even though we were moving quickly. I tried to hang on to consciousness as we sped along the highway. I think I was drifting in and out when we pulled up in front of the entrance.

"Oh no!" said Bruce.

The cleaner was mopping the floors and pointed to the other entrance, so he had to drive around to find a place to park. He quickly helped me inside where a woman was sitting behind a desk. The last thing I remember was Bruce and the woman holding me up as we made our way along the corridor. He told me later that I suddenly stopped in my tracks and slowly sank to the floor.

Bruce told me later that they pumped my stomach and I remained unconscious for twenty-four hours. I could hardly believe it. I felt so ashamed on the day of my departure when the doctor scolded me.

"You have two children, you could have died!"

It only made me feel terribly guilty, which didn't help. He called a few days later, but there was no more communication from the hospital after that except when a social worker came by once shortly afterwards. She suggested I try some artistic outlets to deal with my need for communication, and she pointed out that Bruce and I likely have a communication problem.

I decided to join some classes for sculpting classes, and we worked on our communication. We seemed to be not too bad for awhile. However, the exterior of our house still had to be finished and that took up so much of our time and energy that by the time we were settling down for the night, our effort to communicate slowly fell by the wayside.

Chapter 15

We had been living in our new home for two months in that year of 1977 when out of nowhere I had this strong urge to start on some kind of a spiritual path. It began with a simple question that arose in my mind one day:

What is this soul that we have inside of us?

I remember learning at church that we have a soul, but it was just a word to me for so long. *So what exactly is it?* I wondered.

A few days later while preparing supper for the family, I saw this image on TV where a young woman was sitting in meditation. I was busy at the time so didn't stop what I was doing, but it left me with a desire to find out more. About a week later, I found myself skimming through the *Montreal Gazette* for advertisements relating to yoga meditation and came across a tiny ad that offered classes in Montreal free of charge. I figured I'd try that one first instead of the large ad next to it which had a picture of a bearded guru. The smaller ad read "Ananda Marga offers free personal instruction in yoga meditation." When I called the number, a female voice answered.

"Could I speak with Ananda please?"

I pictured an Indian woman dressed in a traditional sari.

She replied, "Ananda Marga is actually the name of the organization that is offering this course."

It was rather comical, and she gave me information regarding the classes and where to go for the course. Finding this spiritual path was definitely a milestone in my life. I learned the ancient spiritual practices of tantric yoga meditation, which are the tools, so to speak, to be able to delve within one's self to find this soul I had been curious about. I understood that whenever someone has a thirst for any kind of spiritual progress, one will be guided to the right connection in order to move forward. "Knock and the door will open," as Christ said.

After the six-week course, I was initiated by a nun named Didi Uma on October 4, 1977. This is considered to be my spiritual birthday, by the way; it's the day I learned my own personal mantra, which is given according to one's individual vibration. Along with the mantra, I was given my spiritual name, Eta Purna, which means "one who is infinite shining with many colours." I loved the name and was happy to have received personal instruction from her on that very special day.

There are many types of yoga. When we begin doing this tantric meditation, we use a Sanskrit mantra given to us (after we are initiated) by one of the acaryas (monks and nuns) of Ananda Marga. Gradually and with regular practice, the mind evolves from crude to subtle and we become more aware of our soul deep within. This eternal light is actually our witnessing entity to all of our mind's thoughts, words and actions. With the repetition of our mantra, the spiritual energy which is sleeping near the tip of the spine is awakened. Once activated, it begins to move upward along the spinal column, both elevating and purifying the mind at the same time.

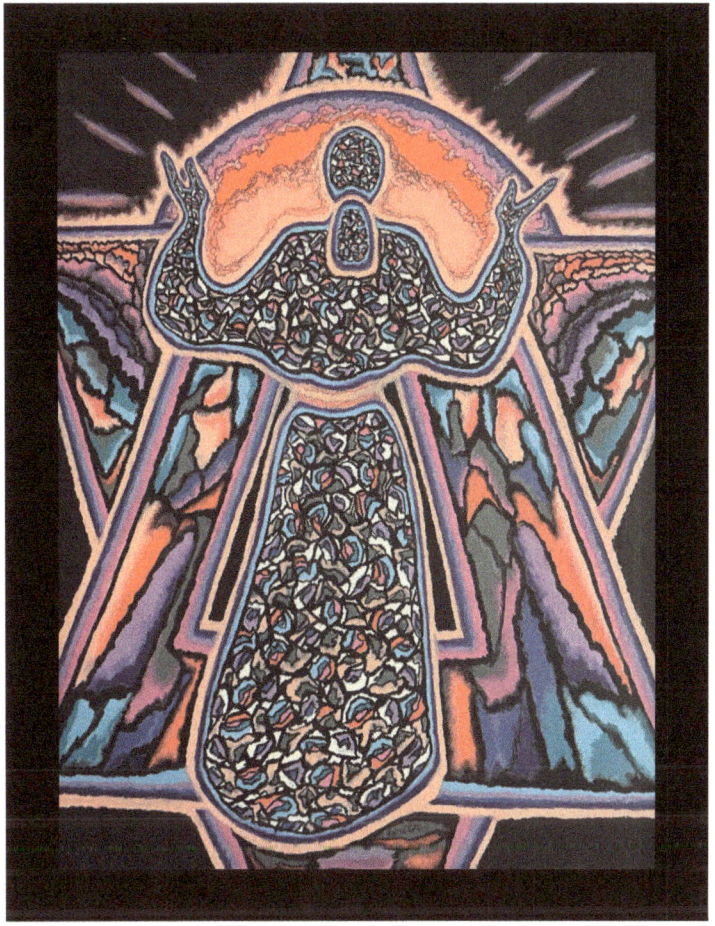

SPIRITUAL DAWN
During the ancient spiritual dance of KIIRTAN- powerful spiritual energy is generated as depicted inside the two triangles - one pointing upwards, the other pointing down.

Also as part of our spiritual practices, our guru passed an ancient spiritual dance, called Akhanda Kiirtan, on to us. It was given over seven thousand years ago by Parvati, the wife of Lord Shiva. In this sacred dance, the spiritual aspirants move together in a circle while singing the universal mantra Baba Nam Kevalam, creating a powerful spiritual energy that is projected outwards into the universe.

In addition to the meditation techniques and ancient spiritual dance Akhanda Kiirtan, we learned ten fundamental principles to follow called Yama and Niyama. Somewhat like the ten commandments, they are the foundation of our spiritual practices. Our guru has emphasized that without these moral principles, spiritual progress is an impossibility.

The five principles of Yama help us to achieve a positive sense of balance in our dealings with society. They are:

Yama

Ahim'sa': Non-injury to others by thought, word or action.

Satya: Action of mind with the right use of words and the spirit of welfare.

Asteya: Not to take possession of what belongs to others, or by omission deprive others of their due.

Aparigraha: To limit our consumption of resources out respect for the common ecological heritage of humanity.

Brahmacharya: To remain attached to Brahma the Supreme Consciousness. To treat the different material objects with which one comes into contact as the different expressions of Brahma, not as the crude formation.

The five principles of Niyama deal more with our personal integration than with our relations to society.

Niyama

Shaoca: Purity and cleanliness, both physical and mental.

Santoṣ'a: Mental contentment along with the sincere effort to evolve in all spheres of life—physical, mental, spiritual

Tapha: Penance by means of rendering service to those less developed or less fortunate than oneself.

Sva'dhya'ya: Clear understanding of the underlying significance of any spiritual subject through proper understanding of their scriptures—all books which help one in mental and spiritual elevation.

Iisvara Pran'idha'na: To accept God as the sole idea of life and to move with accelerated speed towards that supreme shelter.

These moral principles are like guiding posts along this path. They are extremely important in the life of a spiritual aspirant.

I actually had the opportunity to be with our guru Shrii Shrii Anandamurti for the first time in September of 1979 when I attended a global conference and retreat in Jamaica. There was so much excitement with hundreds of margiis arriving from different parts of the world. "Margii" is the name for those initiated into the worldwide spiritual and social service organization of Ananda Marga. The acaryas are the ordained monks and nuns that are from different backgrounds and countries around the world. A female acarya is called a "didi," meaning "sister," and a male acarya is called a "dada," meaning "brother." When we landed in Jamaica, a didi greeted us sisters and a dada greeted the brothers and helped us all get settled in.

Many of the margiis had already been with our guru in India, but this was a first for me. I never did go to India. I was among the dozen sisters who volunteered to learn how to do a new dance our guru had just given while in Jamaica. It was meant for the sisters to perform but brothers may do it as well. This dance called kaoshiki is done with arms reaching straight up over the head and palms touching together while stepping back and forth bending from side to side. It is supposed to make the spine flexible while massaging all the internal organs and helping to maintain good physical health.

A didi showed us how to put on the Indian sari we would wear the next day while dancing kaoshiki in front of our guru in the auditorium. The brothers had their own dance to perform as well, called tandava. It's a rather strenuous ancient dance were they actually hold a large torch in one hand while kicking their legs up as high as they can. I happened to see a couple of brothers demonstrate this dance beforehand without the torch; quite impressive.

The next day, we all gathered in the auditorium where our guru was to deliver his discourse followed by us sisters performing the kaoshiki. The energy was uplifting and inspiring as we swayed in unison in front of our guru and all the margiis that filled the auditorium on that very special occasion. Then it was time for the margii brothers to perform their tandava. It really was awe-inspiring. I could feel the heat of the flames from the torches as they danced while everyone clapped and chanted "Ta ta! Din din!"

Later in the evening of the last day of his discourse, the guru gave us his blessing in Sanskrit from where he stood on the stage. Everyone was sitting on the floor with legs folded in a meditating position. I clearly remember my eyes closing automatically as he raised his hand to give his blessing. Inside my mind I could see only whiteness, no images at all; it was a sacred moment. There was complete silence as we were all transfixed and absorbing this incredibly powerful energy which engulfed the entire auditorium.

Suddenly I felt something brush against my arm. I opened my eyes to see a sister who was sitting on my right fall over onto the floor as if in some kind of a trance. My eye also caught someone on the other side of the auditorium where the brothers were sitting fall over, then maybe one or two more after that.

My understanding is that our guru took onto himself some of their suffering to help lighten their load of samskaras that had accumulated over many lifetimes. A samskara is the potential reaction to a past action. I gazed around in astonishment, taking in all that was unfolding before me, when the silence was suddenly broken with these words from our guru, "Don't become attached to my physical body following me around the globe, go within. I am there."

Each word took hold in my mind as if the message was meant for me alone. The funny thing about that was I never felt the need to follow him around or to go to India as many margiis did. I was quite satisfied doing my spiritual practices regularly at home while taking care of the family. I understood from the beginning that spiritual practices were necessary to take my mind inward on this spiritual journey and that I'd need guidance from the guru. So it resonated on a deep level when he said, "Go within." He simply reaffirmed what I already knew intuitively. I was content to continue on with my spiritual practices as I had been doing while keeping his parting message in the back of my mind.

I received a flyer in the mail with the upcoming retreats and seminars every once in a while, so after attending that special one in Jamaica, I decided to fly to one that was held in Mexico in 1982.

I had become quite good at the bongo drums by playing at home to music on the radio, so I started to play for our akhanda kiirtan events and I took them with me to Mexico. I was glad I did because the margiis were quite happy when I joined in on the akhanda kiirtan there.

While moving in the huge circle of at least sixty margiis and singing our universal mantra Baba Nam Kevalam, a senior monk standing off to my right suddenly caught my attention. His arm was reaching out in my direction just as I was about to pass in front of him, but I assumed he was trying to connect with someone else behind, so I didn't respond. But then he reached in farther, indicating it was me he motioning to, so I stopped playing the drum and stepped away from the circle somewhat puzzled.

As I did, he handed me a tiny piece of paper. The music was quite loud, so it was difficult to hear what he said.

"What's this?" I asked with a raised voice.

He leaned forward to catch my ear and said, "This is your new spiritual name, Amrta."

"But I already have a spiritual name," I said as I glanced at what he had written on the paper.

When he saw I was having trouble pronouncing it, he said, "You can put an 'i' in between the 'r' and 't' if you'd like. The meaning of 'Amrta' is 'a drop of nectar;' look it up to find out more."

After a few tries, I was able to pronounce it properly and thought maybe I should keep it after all. Later, I read that this drop of nectar is secreted by the pineal gland while one is in deep sadhna (an advanced form of meditation). So it is quite special, and I must say I am thankful to have received it.

At the same time, I was happy to keep the name Eta Purna because the didi who initiated me and gave me this name had self-immolated, believe it or not, only a few months after. When I got the news I was stunned, saddened, and confused. She was such a sweet gentle soul. I was totally unaware, of course, that this was going to happen when I dropped her off at the bus station outside of Montreal where we said our final goodbyes.

There is a whole story regarding several monks and nuns who did this. I never had much interest in the political side of the organization as I was drawn only to the spiritual practices. Whenever I connected with the monks and nuns, I was always more comfortable in the company of those who had expressed more devotional sentiment. But then that was just me. Others were open to all aspects of the organization, of course, and they were aware of what was happening on the political level in India.

My understanding of what motivated didi Uma and the others (I believe there were seven altogether) to self-immolate was because our guru, Shrii Shrii Anandamurti, had been imprisoned by Prime Minister Indira Gandhi in the late 1970s and this was their way of protesting. He was actually released and that's why I was able to see him at the conference/retreat in Jamaica in 1979. There were a large number of margiis living in the United States and he had wanted to go there, I was told, but because of the political turmoil at that time, he was denied entry. This left many devotees across the US disappointed with that outcome.

While at the Mexico retreat, I stayed in one of the little cabins with another margii. When we were getting ready for the evening program in the large hall close by, I hesitated for a moment, holding my eyeglasses in one hand and my money in the other.

"Hum, I'm not sure just where I should keep my money," I said. "Maybe I'll just stuff the bills inside my eyeglass case and take it with me to the hall and leave my purse here."

I didn't want to lose it because it was enough for my plane ticket back home.

When I entered the hall, I chose a spot where I could sit down on a cushion on the floor and lean against the wall if necessary during the lecture. I know I put my eyeglass case down on the floor between me and the wall thinking it would be a safe place. I recall telling myself not to forget about it when leaving the hall as well.

I was back in the cabin getting ready for bed when I realized I had left it there, so I rushed over to the hall only to find a couple of people ready to close up for the night. Nothing had been found. I was distraught and didn't know how to handle this problem. The next morning I spoke to one of the acaryas in charge. He surmised that someone cleaning the hall could have conceivably picked it up and that he would do his best to help me out of this tight spot.

When I called Bruce to let him know what was happening, he reassured me that he'd get some money to me so I could fly back home. But time was passing quickly and nothing was being solved. I felt stranded on that last day as everyone was busy packing up to leave. A moment stands out in my mind where I was sitting in the large hall next to the exit kind of staring out at everyone with a blank expression on my face and wondering what to do. They were all preoccupied with organizing their connections, of course, and I was beginning to think I might be left behind. Just then, the dada I spoke to earlier spotted me and looked rather concerned.

"Did you talk to any of the didis about what happened?" he asked.

"No, since you were in charge, I was waiting to see what you could do."

"Okay, stay here, I am going to speak to the senior dada about taking you back with us to our head office in Denver."

I wasn't sure what he meant, but I did as he directed and waited patiently, wanting something—anything—to happen to solve this problem. I was the only one left in the hall with my baggage sitting next to me when the same dada pulled up to the door in a car with a few other dadas inside. One got out and told me I would be going back with them as he put my overnight bag into the trunk of the car.

"Are you sure there's room for me?" I asked.

He just nodded and told me to get in, so I got into the back with two other dadas from India. I sat quietly, concentrating on my mantra while they were kept busy making out their daily reports. As we were about to enter the highway, the dada from the Netherlands who was driving stopped the car and told me to change places with the dada in the back; he wanted me to sit in the passenger's seat instead. I was relieved because it really was uncomfortable with not enough room in the back. I had no idea how long it would take to drive from Monterrey, Mexico, to Denver. I dozed off and woke up when they were changing drivers. It was dark by then.

"Where are we?" I asked.

Someone answered, "We're in Texas, and we'll be driving through this state most of the night."

When we arrived in Denver, the centre was like a beehive with everyone planning and organizing their days. I spent about an hour there before a didi let me know we'd be leaving again soon. She said I couldn't stay at the Denver centre because it was for the brothers who worked from there, so we would be going to the women's training centre in Wichita, Kansas, instead.

"A margii sister will be coming with her car to pick us up within the hour," she said.

She was a trainer who would be giving a six-week course to those interested in becoming yoga teachers.

When the margii sister picked us up, I couldn't help but be inspired by her enthusiasm and energy. They chatted excitedly about this upcoming training session, and I understood there would be about nine other sisters coming from different states, including a sister from Japan who had been studying English. We would be staying in a large house with didi where she lived while giving theses courses. When I called Bruce again to give him the news of where I would be for the next month and a half, I asked if he would please send me money to cover the cost while I was there.

"Sounds like you're not coming home," he said.

So I had to reassure him that I was definitely coming back, just not yet.

"Well, okay. I will arrange to have the money sent to you there as soon as I can."

I knew he would because he always kept his word. Maybe Bruce thought I was making an excuse to stay away longer because things at home were not going all that well. But I definitely had every intention of coming back. It just turned out that I had more time to spend with the other spiritual aspirants while at the training centre. Of course, Robert and Stephen still needed me at home, so I would be back.

When the three of us arrived in Wichita, I was impressed as we entered the lovely large white house. There was a hint of that scent found in ashrams and I immediately felt the peace and serenity. It was such a welcoming change from the confusion that had taken place as the retreat ended, and by now I, too, was highly anticipating the next six weeks.

First, I noticed how simple and clean the rooms were; there was practically no furniture. In the large, bright living room there was a puja table holding the picture of our guru, some candles and a vase of fresh flowers didi brought. A large African drum and other musical instruments sat beside the puja table. The spiritual vibration when we entered was so welcoming, and I couldn't help but feel at ease and inspired to take part in what promised to be a wonderful experience in the weeks ahead.

As didi showed us the five bedrooms we'd be sharing with the other margiis, I noticed a few thin sponges rolled up in the corner and asked about them. She explained that the monks, nuns and trainees don't sleep in beds. They use their sleeping bags, and if they wish, they could put one of those sponges underneath. That was okay with me.

She told us the schedule for the evening and then made some phone calls while the margii sister prepared vegetables for our evening meal. I decided to sit in meditation as I was quite comfortable with the way everything had turned out thus far. Meanwhile, didi was busy receiving incoming margiis and sorting things out for when the course was to begin the next day.

We were up by five the next morning, which is normal for the training sessions, and began each day in the bathroom splashing cool water into the eyes, clearing out the nose and throat using a yoga technique, and splashing water on the glandular system. All of which took only a few second to do. Then we gathered to do the spiritual dance kiirtan for a few minutes before sitting in meditation for half an hour or so. We did our yoga exercises before breakfast and then the scheduled classes for the day began. We did more spiritual practices again before lunch and supper, and the day finally ended with some margiis playing the guitar and singing beautiful devotional songs called bajans that I enjoyed so much. It was a wonderful way to end each day.

Overall, I found the experience at the training centre to be insightful and very interesting. I appreciated not only the knowledge I had gained through the course, but also the wonderful group of sisters I was fortunate enough to connect with on such a deep level while there. I kept in touch with a few of them after returning home, and I was thankful for such a positive experience in Wichita.

Chapter 16

It was March and there was about two feet of snow on the ground when I went to Mexico. I'd expected to return home right after those five days, but by the time I was back home from Wichita in May, the snow had finally disappeared.

When Bruce came to get me at the airport, we were happy to see each other and he seemed interested to hear all about my trip. As we pulled into our yard, I was pleasantly surprised to see Robert and Stephen outside in the yard raking up the leaves. The grass looked so green, and the buds had already opened up on the trees; it felt good to be home again.

I drove to the farm to visit Anita, Janice, Jim and Malcom a couple of days later. Janice was leading her pony out of the barn to get ready for a ride, while Jim and Malcom were farther out in the field. I waved hello and went inside to see if Anita was there. She was standing in front of her easel, focused painting a portrait of a woman. The image she was copying from was pinned up next to the easel.

"Oh, it's you, I'll be with you in a minute," she said.

We hadn't seen each other for a couple of months, so we caught up on the latest on both sides. She never did accept my involvement in Ananda Marga, however, so when I saw she was not interested in what I had to say about my adventures, I kept it short. We mainly talked about her artwork and what I might do the coming summer.

"Why don't you join the Rawdon Artists' Circle?" she said.

This was a group of thirty artists that held yearly exhibitions in a large hall attached to the little United Church in the town of Rawdon, about thirty minutes north of Montreal. I thought about it and decided to give it a try. She showed me how to work with the brush, but it didn't appeal to me, so I opted for oil-based pastels instead. Before I knew it, I had immersed myself in creating colourful expressions and came up with my own technique and style. I liked how it kept my mind so focused, and I would spend a couple of hours almost every day on art. By the time Anita was to have her exhibition, I had a few pieces of my own on display as well.

They always had two exhibitions, one inside and the other outside. We had to send out invitations for the vernissage for the indoor exhibition, which was held one day before the actual sale. Invitees came to have wine and cheese while selecting the art they would like to buy. A small, round, red sticker was placed on the pieces chosen that day. The exhibition was open to the general public the next day to view and purchase what remained.

Each artist had a large display board holding about six paintings, depending on their size. Anita showed some beautiful Rawdon landscapes as well as a couple of portraits. I was a little nervous because my art was so different from the others. They were totally from my imagination, and they expressed emotions relating to my life. One was titled *Yellow Ribbon (tied around the old oak tree)* to welcome the soldiers coming home. Another one, *Tears Of Joy And Sorrow*, show the human eye with a couple of tears falling. They express joy for the soldiers who had returned and sorrow for those who did not. It was a good feeling to have positive feedback from that experience.

The combination of doing artwork and my regular spiritual practices each day helped me become more focused, and I was able to function better than before. That's when I took on a new hobby: making futon mattresses. Our guru had created different departments in the organization, one of which was the Women's Welfare Department (WWD). It was designed to help margii sisters become more independent by earning money from what he said would be a "cottage industry." I saw a documentary on television showing how futons, which were popular at that time, were being made at a factory in Toronto. So I called and they agreed to let me come in person to see how it was done. They were the normal thickness of mattresses, but my thinking was to make my design much thinner so they could be rolled up for travelling to retreats (or anywhere, really). I also hoped to make some money on them.

To make a long story short, I made the thin (2.5 in.) mattresses with beautiful covers and ties to roll them up, and I am proud to say there were of real quality. I put a few in the natural food store in downtown Montreal and they sold. However, for the lack of marketing skills, I never did make any money.

When I saw Anita that fall after I had spent the whole summer working on this project above our two-car garage, she remarked, "You look like a skeleton!" She was right. I'd dropped from my normal, steady weight of 115 lb. to a mere 95 lb. I concluded that not only did I lose weight that summer, but a lot of my time and energy as well, so I simply let go of anymore thoughts of earning money. I ended up giving away my lovely mattresses and meditation cushions to some of the margiis. So much for that endeavour!

In May of 1984, I received a phone call from my sister Yvonne in Toronto telling me that Mama, who was eighty-four years old, had just passed away. I thought I'd take the car and drive to the funeral myself, an eight-hour drive. As I was leaving, Bruce said, "I don't feel comfortable with you going in this old Gremlin, it's not in very good condition!" But I decided to go anyway.

When I arrived, most of the family members were already there in Yvonne's apartment. She was busy in the kitchen, so I didn't want to disturb her. I found a chair in the corner of the living room and sat down by myself. I couldn't help but overhear bits of conversation about Mama's brother, Stephen McLeod, who was only forty-two years old when he died. He had his PhD and was teaching at the University of Montreal when he suddenly had a heart attack in class right there in front of his students. I remembered what they were talking about even though I was only about five years old when it happened.

Their conversations were mainly about members of the family who were considered successful in life (having earned degrees or whatever), and it brought to mind the times when Mama used to compare Anita and I to those who had been educated. Reverting back to those times in my mind, I started to feel a little out of place. Especially when my older brother Junior, who was a sergeant major in the army, spotted me. Everyone was in their Sunday best, so to speak, but there I was wearing a long skirt I had made myself, with my hair pulled back in a plain, earthy look I had taken on when I was first initiated.

As Junior approached with his usual mocking attitude, he said, "Well, look at you, sitting there so demurely all by yourself."

I actually began to tremble slightly inside. *Oh, just ignore him; he hasn't changed*, I told myself. He always delighted in making remarks to intimidate. Sure enough, when he noticed the symbol of our organization on a chain around my neck, he pointed to it and asked, "What's that?" When I told him, he snickered and said, "That's for uneducated people." I simply closed my eyes and internally began repeating my mantra. It actually helped me to disconnect from him altogether.

They didn't understand my yoga lifestyle or my perspective on life itself, so I'm sure they thought I was a little weird. As I got up to go to the kitchen where Yvonne was, Mama's sister, Sister Marion James, reached out to say hello. She was actually a sweet person, but as she turned to walk away, she whispered, "You know, you twins could have gone a long way if only you had finished your education." I'm certain she did not realize how disparaging those remarks were.

It reminded me of when Mama said, "I'm disappointed with the twins" to Louis one time when he was visiting her in Toronto. She was referring to the fact that not only did we not get our education, but Anita and I had been divorced. Back then, there was a stigma attached to those who were separated or divorced. I thought I had forgotten all those negative remarks about us, but it wasn't so. Being with them even for that short time made me see how much I had changed over the years. At least now I understood where they were coming from—it was no different from when we were growing up.

As I looked around, I couldn't help but notice that Anita and Adeline were absent but Justine was there. Actually there were quite a few family members missing. Later on when I mentioned this to Adeline, she said matter-of-factly, "Why should I go? Mama never loved us!" She said that one night when she came home late, Mama beat her with a stick across the back of her legs as she ran upstairs to get away.

"It didn't matter that I was already engaged to Wilfred, who I had been out with that night," said Adeline.

That's when it dawned on me that Anita and I were not the only ones with bad memories of living at home. But since none of them ever talked about it, I never knew. Of course, I already knew how Anita felt and definitely understood why she had stayed away. I have to admit that deep down I really did not want to go either, but I felt obligated for some reason.

At the funeral procession, I happened to be sitting in a car next to Yvonne's daughter, and as our long line of cars slowly passed through the gate of the cemetery, she quipped, "Oh come on, Granny! Why did you pick your plot so far in the back? It's taking us forever to get there." She said it so innocently, and we couldn't help but laugh.

I left for home right after the casket was lowered into the ground. Memories of how we were raised in New Waterford, being left in Montreal—basically our lives in general, and well, just life and death itself—flooded my mind. The memory of having come so close to dying a few years back after swallowing those pills was sobering. I would normally have the radio tuned to upbeat music when driving alone, but not today. I contemplated my behaviour and why I reacted the way I did. In doing so, I understood myself a little more and why I had turned out the way I did. That goes for Anita as well, since we were both in the same boat, so to speak, from day one.

That long ride home by myself gave me plenty of time to mull over what I had forgotten regarding family relationships. I became very emotional at one point, sincerely wanting to forgive those who had hurt me, but I quickly realized I had to start with myself. I had to forgive myself for the pain I had caused others. I must say, this helped to pacify my mind quite a bit.

At the same time, though, I was worried about my future with Bruce. I also thought about the fact that Robert and Stephen would not need me much longer. As these thoughts were passing through my mind, my attention suddenly shifted to my car; it wasn't responding the way it should. I was driving along the 401 Expressway, the corridor between Toronto and Montreal, and noticed that when I pressed on the gas pedal it did not gain any speed. *That's strange,* I thought. I did not want to stop because I thought it was too dangerous with the heavy traffic. When I saw the sign Brockville, I immediately took that exit.

But oh dear!—the car did not respond at all when I pressed on the gas. In fact it slowed down! I'd have to pull off to the side as far as possible while it was still rolling to a stop- right there on the exit ramp!

Holy God, NO! Don't stop here!

Other vehicles were following behind with their flashers indicating they were about to exit the expressway right behind me. I wasn't quite off the shoulder when the first one, a large truck, whizzed by. The wind jolted my car and made me nervous. I carefully opened the door and edged my way around to open the hood. It was too hot to the touch, and steam started to come out from underneath.

The next vehicle coming along the ramp was a pickup truck, so I waved it down. The young man opened the hood and said, "I think you'll need a tow truck; looks like the problem is in the motor. I'll take you to a garage just down the road if you want."

"Oh thank you so much!" I said as I climbed into his pickup. "I was on my way to Ottawa, but now it looks like I'll have to take the bus from here."

"I will show you where the bus station is on our way to the garage," he said.

It just happened to be where the margii family lived, so I figured I could stay there overnight and continue on to Saint-Jean-de-Matha the next day. At the garage I was told Ottawa was only forty-five minutes away, and after giving them the information they needed, I was dropped off at the bus station nearby.

I connected with the margii family in Ottawa and stayed the night, and I was on the bus for home the next morning. Meanwhile, Bruce had to deal with our car situation. I was remorseful by now, remembering what he had said about not being comfortable with me taking the car. I really should have listened to him.

By the time I reached home I had already sorted out a number of things I would have done differently if I had the chance. With nothing but good intentions, I was ready to make changes for the better. I knew I had to if Bruce and I were to stay together. It dawned on me that whenever I decided to do something, there was no stopping me. I ignored any red flags and just went ahead with whatever; there was no rational thinking. I really needed to stop doing that. I wanted to think twice before moving too quickly on whatever it was I decided to do from then on.

Meantime, because Anita and I had not been in touch for a while, I was not aware she had been thinking about leaving the farm when Janice was ready to go to college. I knew that Malcom had never accepted Anita and that their marriage had been on shaky ground for quite a while, so I wasn't too surprised when I heard they had separated. She had taken a room in Grey Manor, she told me, a boarding house on the main street in Rawdon. The elderly lady who was president of the artists' circle owned and operated the manor, and being a retired nurse, she also took care of a couple of the residents.

After living there for a few months, Anita found a small bungalow within walking distance to the little church, and she joined the choir. Not long after that, she told me she had met someone and decided to marry again, this time it was a man around her own age. His name was George, and he was a long-distance truck driver who made regular trips back and forth to the United States.

I had not seen Anita since I came back from mama's funeral, which was in May, so I thought it was about time to visit her. It was a cold winter day just a few days after a huge snowstorm. George was home with her at the time, and we got to know each other a little before I noticed it was starting to get dark outside, so I decided to leave.

I was a little uneasy since the roads were not in the best condition. The drive over was a bit slippery in spots, which made it dangerous to drive, especially at night. We were standing at the door in their kitchen while saying our goodbyes when I happened to look out the kitchen window and saw what looked like flames pouring out of their neighbour's upstairs window.

"OH MY GOD!" I gasped, "IS THAT FIRE I SEE COMING OUT OF LUCY'S WINDOW?"

Lucy and her husband were an elderly couple from Italy. Fortunately, I already had my jacket and boots on, so I sprang into action. I bolted out the door, grabbing onto the railing as I almost slipped rushing down the steps. The snow had been plowed in the driveway, so I was able to run across to reach the fence that was between the two houses.

When I got to the gate, the snow on the other side made it almost impossible to push it open, but somehow I managed to squeeze through. The snow was knee deep, which slowed me down.

The kitchen door was wide open, and I rushed inside to see Lucy frantically grabbing a few things as if wanting to take them with her. A thin veil of smoke slowly drifted around the room. Marco was lying face down on the kitchen floor a few feet in front of me! Apparently he was trying to put the flames out because a bucket was overturned on the floor next to him. My mind jumped into overdrive.

"LUCY! WHAT ARE YOU DOING?" I shouted. "LEAVE THAT AND GET OUT!"

She dropped the toaster she was holding, reached up to unhook a cage holding two white doves and staggered out the door with it. I couldn't tell whether her husband was still alive, but his eyes were closed. I am no paramedic and wasn't about to determine his condition, so I tried to pull him towards the door, but he was dead weight. *I don't think he's alive!* I thought, so I ran out the door to get help.

I caught up with Lucy as she struggled through the deep snow without any coat or boots on. She was hanging onto the cage with the doves inside, one of which escaped when the door suddenly flew open. I was able to slam the cage shut and prevent the other one from flying off. I was afraid Marco would be engulfed in the flames which were spreading quickly, so I turned and headed back to the house to get him.

As I did, what looked like a black wire suddenly snapped and flung into the air with sparks flying everywhere, giving me quite a scare. In that second with a bit of light from the sparks, I saw a few people standing nearby looking on. I spotted George, so I kept on moving towards the house, but when I glanced back to see if he was coming, he'd suddenly stopped in his tracks as if not sure what to do next.

"COME ON!" I shouted "WE HAVE TO GET HIM OUT!"

When we reached the kitchen door, the roaring from the fire upstairs was much louder—and terribly frightening indeed! I tried not to panic so I could focus on getting Marco out of the house. Some sparks falling from the upstairs window landed on my cloth coat as we struggled to get him through the door and down the back steps. We had trouble hanging onto him once we started trudging through the knee-deep snow as well.

I don't know how we ever managed to squeeze through the gate while carrying him, but we finally made it to Anita's house where we placed him on the couch in her living room. Lucy was in a state of shock. She was standing in front of the picture window and asking (as if talking to herself), "Where's the Red Cross? Where's the Red Cross?"

The firefighters and paramedics arrived, and they confirmed that Marco had already passed away. Lucy said he had been running up and down the stairs with buckets of water to put the flames out in the chimney upstairs where it started. He suddenly collapsed on the kitchen floor just before I entered the house.

A TV news crew showed up at the door asking if someone would say something regarding the tragedy that had just unfolded. When I agreed, a small mic was clipped onto my sweater and I said a few words. Unfortunately, the firemen, who were all volunteers, were not able to get there in time, so after the flames were extinguished, the house was declared a total loss.

Lucy was taken to her son and daughter in-law's home in a suburb of Montreal. I went to see her shortly afterwards. While there I found out she was about to become a grandmother for the very first time to twin girls! I was so happy for her, and we did keep in touch with short visits for a few years after that.

Being at home taking care of the household and doing my spiritual practices was a simple lifestyle that I needed because of the chronic pain I had been living with for many years. I finally saw a good naturopathic doctor in Montreal who was able to diagnose the underlying cause of my pain. It stemmed from the back injury I sustained when the steering wheel hit my back in that car crash back in 1964.

"Your back really should have been looked at immediately after that accident," he said. "Your spine has endured too much over the years, and you have a herniated disc between the sixth and seventh vertebrae in the neck and a problem at the joint in your left hip. Unfortunately, your spine will need as much time to heal as it did to deteriorate. But you do have one thing in your favour," he added, "and that's the healthy lifestyle you've described living, with regular yoga exercises and proper diet."

Accepting the fact that this would be a long and tedious process, I began chiropractic treatments every two weeks. I continued with my yoga exercises and meditation every morning to maintain an all-round healthy lifestyle. Not only are the muscles stretched while putting pressure on the glands and releasing hormones into the blood stream during yoga, but the massage we did at the end touches all the reflex points, leaving both body and mind feeling balanced and totally relaxed.

I also became a vegetarian when I was initiated, and I really got into cooking at that time. Using the soybean as a base, I made vegetarian burgers that everyone liked, thick spaghetti sauces and even home-made tofu, yogurt and sprouted alfalfa seeds. Some dishes the family liked and some not so much. I tried to keep the meals close to what we ate before my switch.

Aside from this change in diet, there were other significant changes as well. For example, whenever I received a flyer in the mail for upcoming retreats that were held about every six months, I always had that to look forward to. Each time before I left, I made sure I cooked enough food to put into the freezer for the family while I was away.

Every once in a while, I'd get a call from one of the acaryas as he or she passed through Montreal. I'd pick them up at the bus, train or airport, depending on where they were coming from. They stayed in my home for a couple of days after the apartment they had used as a meditation centre when I was initiated was no longer available.

The young lady who was giving the course in meditation at that time decided to go to India to become an acarya. After that, us local margiis got together in each others' homes for our dharmachakra (a gathering for collective meditation). About a dozen of us would come together to have our kiirtan and meditation, followed by a vegetarian pot luck. We enjoyed sharing the interesting experiences we'd had, especially with those who had personal contacts with our guru Shrii Anandamurti while they were in India.

Shortly after the retreats in Jamaica and Mexico, I flew down to one in the southern United States. I forget exactly where it was, but it was in the mid 1980s. There were a large number of margiis, and there is one that stands out in my mind that I cannot forget. His name was Wil Nolan and he came from California. He was a talented musician and a great devotee of the Supreme. I was struck by his deep devotion which he expressed so beautifully in the songs he had composed and recorded. I was captivated as I sat there listening to his soft voice singing words that held such depth and understanding of our connection to the Supreme. Just before we were to leave the retreat, he personally handed me a tape of his recording *Crystal Sun*, which I now have on a CD. I also have *Remembering Ba Ba* that he had recorded after our guru passed away in 1990. Even now, decades later, his words still have a way of reaching out to me and are as fresh and inspirational today as they were when I first heard them.

There was an Ananda Marga retreat held every year in Missouri that I wanted to attend because they had a large piece of property out in the country called a master unit. I decided to drive instead of flying, and there was an acarya who had stayed at my place a number of times who mentioned he, too, was interested in going to that retreat. His name was dada Rainjit, a young blond dada from Norway. He happened to be in Toronto at the time, so I figured I'd first drive the eight hours there, pick him up and continue on from there.

However, there were a couple of unexpected obstacles we had to face once we started our journey. One was the weather. We had a heatwave to contend with, and my old gremlin did not have air-conditioning. I couldn't cope physically by the time we reached Indiana, I think it was, when the extreme heat became too much, so dada had to take over the driving for me. At one point we had to stop along the highway so I could throw up next to the car. I also had terrible pain in my head.

We decided to stop at the nearest motel on the highway where he slept in the car and I spent the night in the motel. Next morning when I felt well enough to continue, he advised, "You should see a homeopathic doctor when you get back home; your thermostat seems to be broken."

He mentioned that he had been studying to be a doctor before he decided to become an acarya.

When we finally arrived at the retreat, I was in pretty bad shape. I went to lie down with the intention of taking part in the meditation program later on that evening. I was not able to get up again until the next morning when everyone was about to go see the waterfalls nearby, so I went along. It was still baking hot, and I started to think I shouldn't have gone with them after all.

By the time we got back, I was once again feeling overwhelmed from the heat. As we entered the building I stumbled and someone had to catch me. Fortunately, there was a nurse among us who took over and attended to my needs right away. She said I was likely suffering from heat exhaustion.

I don't remember much about the retreat itself. Needless to say, both dada and I were more than happy when we finally reached Toronto. I stayed at Yvonne's place until I was strong enough to drive back home, and I vowed to never tackle a long-distance drive like that again.

Afterwards, I made a point of going to retreats and seminars that were close to home. I enjoyed driving down through the Adirondack Mountains when the trees were changing colours in the fall in New York State and Vermont. Eventually, I chose smaller retreats that were even closer to home, like Ottawa, where I got to know margiis Chris and Jane quite well and felt comfortable staying in their home over the weekend when they organized little retreats for us.

At home, I always went out into the fields, which took only a couple of minutes to reach from our house, to sit in meditation all by myself. I loved the peace and quiet there. Surrounded by the rolling hills of the Canadian shield and away from any sound of traffic, I was able to spend time undisturbed doing my spiritual practices during the warm weather. I felt blessed and thankful to be there.

Robert and Stephen loved to ride on the trails. Stephen on his dirt bike and Robert on his expensive mountain bike made to tackle the steep slopes where professional bikers often competed. One time Stephen asked me if I would like to go for a ride on a four-wheeler through the fields near our home. I am sure he was trying to scare me by the way he was swerving carelessly up and down the little hills. I did my best to hang on, refusing to let him see just how frightened I was. He thought it was funny, but I didn't; it was extremely dangerous. Anyway, I never did get back on that four-wheeler again. I simply did not trust his judgment or understand his sense of humour.

By the time they had reached their teens, their interest naturally turned to cars, although they still liked to ride on the trails near home. In the winter, Robert often went to the higher Laurentian Mountains nearby, where he enjoyed skiing the slopes with a few of his friends.

Around the time when Bruce went from being hatchery manager in the village of Saint-Félix-de-Valois where they hatched baby chicks in incubators, to managing a large turkey farm out on the highway, Robert turned fifteen years old. He wanted to earn some money, so Bruce gave him work on the farm during summer vacation. The following summer he got a job working in a printing shop in our little town of Saint-Jean-de-Matha where he learned the graphic arts trade.

Meanwhile, Bruce and I were more or less going through the motions of daily life. Every once in a while, because of some misunderstanding in communication between us, I suffered from what I found out later to be "triggers." This happened whenever I had a wrong perception, where I believed I was being rejected, or simply being ignored when I needed to be heard. When this occurred, I was never able to comprehend what was happening to me or why I was getting so upset.

For example, one day Bruce and I happened to be in Ottawa, which is about a three-and-a-half-hour drive from home. I recall wanting to go to the National Gallery there to see the beautiful paintings of Tom Thomson and The Group of Seven. I don't remember what we were talking about as we walked towards the gallery, but something Bruce said suddenly triggered a feeling of disconnect where I had this wrong perception that he didn't want to be with me.

With this thought in mind, everything turned upside down for me. I only remember reacting as I always did when I believed I was being rejected: I became upset and started to cry. It was bad enough when this happened when we were at home, but now here we were in a public place! I was never able to control my emotions once I was triggered and was completely devoid of any rational thought, which made it even more difficult to deal with.

As we approached the elevator in the gallery, the door opened and a young lady in uniform who obviously worked there stepped out holding a pager in her hand. She took a few steps, stopped, and looked at me as if wondering what happened. When she saw I was trying to avoid eye contact with her (I was terribly embarrassed to been seen in this state), she asked, "Madam, are you okay? Do you want me to call security?" Bruce was alarmed when she said this and started to back away as if he thought he might get into trouble if he stayed.

"It's okay, there's no problem," I said to her, wanting to minimize what might have appeared to be more serious than it really was.

To divert attention away from myself, I quickly stepped into the elevator when the light turned green and it took me up to the main floor. In doing so, I momentarily lost track of Bruce and the lady in uniform. When I returned to the basement, neither one of them were in sight. This caused a lapse of judgment in my mind where I actually believed Bruce had "intentionally" left me there alone. Becoming more anxious by the minute, I began wandering around the parking lot searching for our white Toyota. *Where could he be?* I felt as if I was about to panic when I suddenly spotted our car, which was still parked where we had left it.

I expected to see Bruce when I approached, but he was nowhere to be found. Holding back tears of frustration, I stood next to the car and carefully scanned the parking lot. *God! Where could he be?* I wondered. Just then I remembered he had given me the keys for safekeeping while we were walking towards the elevator. Thankfully, there they were in my purse, so I opened the door and sat inside where I tried to calm down.

For the life of me I could not understand what was happening. I was exasperated to the point where I just wanted to give up and go home—with or without him. The longer I sat there thinking about it, the more impatient I became.

The next thing I remember is starting the car and slowly driving around the parking lot, straining anxiously to see if he might still be around. But when I had reached the exit out of the building, I just continued driving. The next thing I knew I was on the route taking me out of Ottawa and onto the highway.

My mind started jumping around with thoughts of what I should have done instead. *Maybe I shouldn't have left?* I questioned whether his leaving me there really did justify my leaving him in turn. By then a mild throbbing pain had started inside my head. I figured it must be from the stress. Whenever I drove to Ottawa by myself I managed the pain by simply stopping periodically along the way to rest. It started even before I was out onto the highway that day, so I braced myself for the drive ahead knowing only too well what I was in for.

Ignoring the pain and determined to get home as soon as possible despite the signals my body was giving me, I continued. Earlier when Bruce and I were on our way to Ottawa, it wasn't necessary for me to stop to rest because he was doing the driving and I was just fine. But now my entire system had been affected. Fortunately, the pillow and sleeping bag I always used when I travelled alone was in the trunk, so I knew I'd have that to rely on if needed.

I know three and a half hours for a trip doesn't sound like much, but when you're dealing with physical pain, it's another matter altogether. I kept on driving until I had passed the three-hour mark and finally I realized I had no choice; I definitely had to stop because the pain had become unbearable. I was approximately twenty minutes away from home when I finally pulled off the expressway into a small rest area.

When I came to a stop in front of the little building on the circular driveway, I noticed there were no other vehicles or people around. I got out and opened the back door to get the special chiropractic pillow I used to support my neck and head whenever I had to stop while travelling. I planned to lie down in the back seat of the car with my sleeping bag and pillow for at least half an hour. But I was in such agony that I didn't even think to be cautious. I just laid down on the park bench right there next to my car. I threw my pillow onto it, then with piercing pain in my head, I slowly tried to find a position comfortable enough to rest for at least ten minutes.

What a tremendous relief to just lie there on my back with the gentle breeze on my aching body. While gazing up at the large green maple leaves hanging overhead and the sun's rays filtering through the branches, I felt thankful I was able to make it this far. But within seconds the words *LEAVE! NOW!* sprung from deep within my mind. Instantly and spontaneously, without any question whatsoever, my entire being responded to this command. I automatically rose up to a sitting position as if being aided by some unseen force. It is rather difficult to describe what occurred at that exact moment because it happened so fast.

As I opened my eyes, I was stunned to see two men moving quickly towards me, both with the look of evil intent on their faces. Within a split second, even in the complete shock of that moment, I was able to capture the entire scene. Directly in front of me, an ominous looking man with dark hair who was probably in his forties was closing in on me. To my right, another man who was around sixty and had thick white hair crept out from behind the trunk of a large tree. He had a strange gleeful expression on his face, as if to say, "We got her!"

Only the length of my car and the bench stood between us. I honestly felt there was no way out. I was absolutely petrified! I knew instinctively that turning and running would be useless because they would catch up to me within seconds. So I had no choice but to make a bold move towards them in order to reach my car which I remembered I did not lock. At the risk of not making it in time, I dashed forward to grab the handle of the car door. I have an indelible image of the look of sheer determination on one of the men's faces as he reached out to grab me; it still sends shivers down my spine. I was only inches away from his grasp, and I managed to open the door and jump inside.

Totally panic-stricken, I turned on the ignition and pressed the gas pedal to the floor. With the high-pitched squeal of the tires in my ears, I barely made it around the circular driveway as I sped onto the expressway without even glancing in the mirror as I merged. I only realized I was safe and out of their reach when I found myself on the highway. I had to slow down to the speed limit.

In utter shock and disbelief, the reality sank in during the rest of my drive home. Obviously, I had been in survival mode while making what I can only describe as a miraculous escape. I say "miraculous" because there is no way I could have avoided being harmed that day if I did not have that warning in my mind at that precise moment. It is a profound experience I will never forget, and it served to deepen my faith and trust that I am always being guided by a higher power.

I should explain here that I believe in the universal law of karma, where our actions, whether good or bad, determine what we have to live through in this lifetime. This is looking at the overall big picture. When we close in on the smaller picture, so to speak, we can see that whatever actions we do today will affect how our day will go tomorrow. I always thought the expression "we reap what we sow" meant literally putting seeds into the earth. Later I realized it's about planting seeds in the mind that eventually sprout when conditions are right in the spiritual realm, where we undergo the reactions, both good and bad. The reality is that nothing is happening at random. As our guru pointed out, "There is no such thing as accident; everything is incident." With my understanding that everything unfolds as it should in this universe, I am able to accept all that is taking place around me and in my own life as well more readily.

When I finally arrived home, the first thing I did was reach for the painkillers. Next, I was on the phone to report the incident to the police. After describing what happened, I said, "So I lost my pillow!"

"You could have lost your life, madam," the officer said. "An elderly gentleman was robbed and murdered there just a few weeks ago."

"Oh no. I was not aware! That easily could have been *my* fate today!" I said.

"So we will get onto this right away, madam. Take care of yourself."

That was the only time I spoke to the police and I never heard anything after that. I must say I have deep sympathy for the elderly gentleman who lost his life there at the rest area, and for every other person undergoing heavy karmic reactions while on this earth. At the same time, I am happy for those reaping the benefits of their good karmic reactions as well.

I do not believe that I was somehow favoured by a higher power when I was spared from the hands of those criminals. As narrow an escape as it was, I simply was not meant to experience the same fate as that poor man. I was able to make it home safely to make that report to the police and was thankful to have another day to get things right in the future as far as my relationship with Bruce was concerned.

As I hung up the phone after giving my report, my mind turned to Bruce. I knew he would be worried once he discovered the car was gone. He probably thought I would be coming back for him at any moment. By that point I regretted leaving Ottawa the way I did that morning. It must have seemed like a very long wait for Bruce.

That day's drama left me totally drained. Finally safe at home after making the call to the police, I flopped down onto my bed. Then the phone rang. It was Bruce! When I heard his voice on the other end exclaiming, "You're home!" I broke down. "Where did you go? I couldn't find you!" I cried. I knew there was nothing I could do to help him at that point and neither of us were in the mood for a lengthy discussion, so he simply said he would come home by bus. I was sleeping like a log by the time he got back.

I do not recall us talking about it the next day, so we must have forgiven each other for the way we both handled the situation. Neither of us had ever played the blame game at least. Instead, we tended to just let go of whatever problem we might have been facing in order to avoid further conflict. We stayed together despite my occasional triggers, which I knew were not easy for him to live with.

I began to wonder what the future held once Robert and Stephen didn't need me anymore. Robert had just turned eighteen, and he decided to pursue his graphic arts training in Montreal. Within a couple of weeks, he found a full-time job in this line of work which he really enjoyed. Before long, he bought himself a brand-new Honda Civic that he took great pride in, washing and polishing it when at home on weekends. Stephen preferred to stay in Saint-Jean-de-Matha and found work fixing computers in Joliette.

As always, Bruce had his own interests that kept him busy outside of work. I, on the other hand, only had connection with the margiis and acaryas. Actually, I remember the last time I got together with them at my place very well because I suffered a trigger on that particular day.

Just after our collective meditation, we sat down for our vegetarian meal. I was quite relaxed and interested in engaging in conversation. When I asked the dada next to me a question and he didn't respond, it instantly changed my entire demeanour. I'd had this issue with him before, but he seemed oblivious to how it affected me. I tried to rise above it this time—after all, it does seem kind of petty and insignificant—but for whatever reason I wasn't able to let it go. In the blink of an eye, I stood up and without thinking blurted out, "Okay, that's it for me!" and began gathering the dishes and placing them in the sink. It stunned everyone, including me.

There was some grumbling among the margiis as they were getting ready to leave, while dada went to the phone to make a call. As he did, he turned to me with a concerned look and said, "You only hurt yourself!" I was unable to control my emotions, and I knew I was in need of some kind of professional help. It was quite disheartening to say the least, especially because I did it within my spiritual group!

I had been struggling for so many years with an inability to fit into any kind of social situation, but that day I was painfully aware of how awful my behaviour had been. I understood I would have to undergo the consequence of my actions. Since this clearly was not working out for me, I thought my decision to disconnect from the organization was the right thing to do. But *not* in the way it happened there at the table with the negative effects it had on everyone!

As usual after a trigger, I broke down and cried. It had been ten years since I was initiated, and now I had to look for other ways to fill the gap I had just created.

Chapter 17

So I started to think in terms of personal relationships and what I might do to find some satisfaction in that arena. I wanted to deepen my understanding of why I was having so much trouble connecting with people because it was taking a toll on my relationship with Bruce as well. We were not as close as I would have liked. I really was perplexed as to what to do about it, since we both seemed to feel stuck with this problem—*my* problem, I should say.

Since Anita had taken the plunge and remarried and was now having what appeared to be a relatively normal life, it made me think I, too, might find someone out there. That maybe, just maybe, I could end up with a soulmate some day.

After pondering this scenario for a while, I mentioned it to Bruce. He wasn't surprised since I had always been like an open book, saying exactly what was on my mind. He knew me much better than I realized because, when I bought a map of Ottawa to memorize the major routes and streets in the downtown area with the idea that I would like to move there, he'd say, "The grass always looks greener on the other side," or "You know you can't live in an apartment there all by yourself!" It made me stop and think, *He's right. What the heck am I doing?* So I'd forget about it for a while, but then something inside made me come back to this idea every once in a while. I couldn't seem to let go of it.

Even though I had disconnected from the organization, I still wanted to maintain the connection I had with the margii family living in Ottawa; I'd never had any problems while in their company. However, the little retreats happened less frequently, so I didn't have anyone to share my spiritual practices with anymore. I'd heard about an organization that held their retreats in the Laurentian Mountains just north of Montreal, so I went there for a weekend. I wasn't familiar with their spiritual practices, so I didn't feel comfortable. It was as if I was in this world but not part of it, if that makes any sense.

Slowly but surely this disconnect began to affect my mental health. I found myself turning to Bruce more often than usual when I felt the need to connect. (By the way, I am not referring to connecting sexually here or any time I write about needing attention.) I'd never had a partner I could connect with on an emotional level. I was considering just giving up altogether because if something didn't change for the better, our future would be unhappy.

One day just before or after Easter Sunday in 1987, I was doing my usual housework and spiritual practices when I decided I wanted to get some fresh air. The meltdown started when I was out walking along our country road close to home. Large, soft snowflakes gently fell all around me, and I was just grateful to be there in that moment and feel some peace and tranquility.

As I was strolling along in that lovely setting with the surrounding hills giving a sense of protection from the world itself, I began to feel a pressure inside my head, not painful, just a sort of tightness. This had occurred a few times before during a real snowstorm, and I'd had a difficult time with the onset of triggers. I began to feel vulnerable and became concerned because I knew how volatile the situation could become if I were to ask Bruce for help. Chances were not very good that he'd be there for me.

When I got back to the house, I was cautiously optimistic as I reached for the phone to call Bruce. He was at his friend's house, and I asked him if he would mind coming home because I needed to talk to him.

"Why are you calling me here?" he asked with a tone that suggested I was intruding; I'd never called him there before.

Not what I needed to hear at that moment. I felt this sickening in the pit of my stomach indicating I was about to suffer another trigger. I had put myself into an extremely vulnerable position once again where I was about to be either ignored or rejected, so I said, "Oh never mind!" and slammed the phone down. My head started to spin with frightful images of how this might play out when he finally did come home. I told myself I was not about to go through that again and definitely did not want him to have to deal with it either!

I realized I needed some kind of help, but I was at a loss as to how to get it. I knew from past experiences that when I had a trigger, I'd most likely end up shouting "Get out!" because I wasn't getting anywhere connection-wise. I also flashed back to the "pill problem," so I was determined to find a solution before it escalated.

So I dialled the police, something I had never done before, hoping they might take me to the hospital in Joliette. There I might be able to find help through their mental health department. I wasn't thinking clearly—I only knew something terrible was about to happen if I did not take action.

So when two French-speaking officers arrived shortly after, I couldn't clearly explain my problem in French. A female officer probably didn't understand my French, so I turned to the male officer and said in English, "I want to get to the hospital in Joliette. I need help. Could you please take me there?"

"No, we don't do that," he said with such a hard look on his face.

I just couldn't hold it together any longer. I pushed him in the chest, causing him to step backwards and almost lose his balance. He grabbed my arm, forcing me to stand still, but then I saw Bruce driving along our street towards our house.

"There's my husband!" I said on the verge of striking out again as I squirmed out of his hold.

Bruce, of course, looked shocked as he pulled into our driveway.

"What's going on?" he asked, getting out of the car.

"I want to go to the hospital in Jolliette, so I asked if they'd take me there but they refused," I said as I hopped into the driver's seat. "But it's okay now; I can drive myself!"

Bruce snatched the keys out of the ignition, telling me to calm down as the officers approached and began speaking to him in French. I couldn't have cared less about whether they understood or not. I needed to speak to a professional who could actually help me.

Bruce opened the passenger side door of our car and told me to get in.

"I'll take you over," he said, knowing full well how unpredictable that ride could be.

To be honest, I was terribly afraid of doing something crazy like jumping out of the car if I freaked out for some reason. I'm not kidding.

We reached the highway a mile and a half away from our house without incident, but then I saw in the rear-view mirror that instead of turning right onto the highway to go back to their station, the police car was now following us. When we arrived at the hospital, the officers came in and spoke to someone who appeared to be in charge. Bruce went to the reception to explain why we were there.

He appeared to be suggesting I might suddenly go crazy and attack someone. It sounded like he said he simply did not know what to do with me. I needed his support, but I felt as if I he barely knew me. This made me more upset and it showed.

Someone took my left arm and Bruce took my right as they walked me down the hallway. I desperately wanted to speak with someone I could feel emotionally safe with and be able to find the help I urgently needed, but it wasn't turning out that way.

I couldn't communicate with anyone, and I started to think it was a mistake to come to the hospital. I was told to change into a hospital gown, and then I was brought into another room that was painted green. There was a long table that had thick leather straps hanging from each side. It's not easy to describe my emotions at that point.

"WHAT? WHAT'S THIS!"

I was furious. Without a word, someone helped me get onto the table, and to my utter dismay, he took one arm and began to strap it down.

"What are you doing!"

I began to struggle, but before I knew it, my other arm was firmly strapped into place. *How can this be happening to me?* I couldn't fathom Bruce actually allowing them to do this! I wanted to scream for help but a wave of calmness swept over me. I instinctively knew that if I panicked while being strapped down, I might pass out. I was already finding it difficult to breath.

I turned my head towards a door with a small window and saw Bruce looking in. Our eyes connected as the nurse stood over me with a large needle in his hand. I was horrified! It must have showed on my face because Bruce stepped inside the room and told him not to administer the shot. This was playing out like some kind of a nightmare!

"Where are my clothes?" I pleaded. "I want to get dressed."

They undid the straps and brought me back to the room where my clothes were. On the night table next to a bed were two white pills and a glass of water. I was told I should take them, which I did.

Dressed and anxious to get out of there, I stepped out into the hallway. As I did, a man probably in his fifties was being led down the corridor with someone on each side of him. It was obvious he did not want to go. They took him into the room where I had been strapped down.

"Oh no, they're going to strap him down!" I said in disbelief.

My heart went out to him as he began to resist at the door. I tried to accept that this procedure must have been designed to be helpful, but surely there had to be some more humane way to handle patients. It really was a terrible, degrading and humiliating experience.

Not much was said on our way back from the hospital; guess we were just relieved that the drama had ended. I always needed at least a couple of days to recover.

I knew for certain that I needed professional help, so I called a medical centre in downtown Montreal and got an appointment the following week. I had to move quickly on this because I didn't know how much longer Bruce and I would stay together.

The doctor told me I had a condition known as bipolar, which is a mood disorder. He pointed to a picture on the wall of a young lady in her graduation outfit holding a degree.

"That's my daughter" he said. "She has the same bipolar condition as you have."

"I knew for a long time that there was something wrong with me," I said. "At least now I know it actually has a name."

Yes, and you will need medication, so I'll give you a prescription that you can have filled here in our building on your way out if you'd like. You'll receive a call for your next appointment with me within a few days."

I did as he said and headed back home to Saint-Jean-de-Matha. Bruce was not at all surprised with the diagnosis and seemed relieved when I showed him the pills I would start taking that night. I actually thought this was going to cure me, and that everything would be just fine from then on.

The first pills made me nauseous and a little dizzy, so I stopped taking them after just a few days. Bruce thought I should continue taking them anyway, but I didn't. I figured I'd tell the doctor about this when I saw him at my next appointment. He wasn't too happy with my decision either.

"Would it be possible to be referred to a psychologist?" I asked.

"If this is what you want," he said. "I can refer you to a colleague in this building."

I was surprised when her office called me the next day and booked an appointment for that week. I had high expectations as I waited outside her office. I hoped we would have a good connection and that the hour of talk therapy scheduled would be a strong start. *This is exactly what I need,* I thought. *I don't want to take any pills if I don't have to.*

She started by asking me questions about my family, how many brothers and sisters did I have, etc. She was listening intently, so I started to feel comfortable with her.

"What kind of a relationship do you have with your father?" she asked.

I told her I thought it was a good one but that he had passed away when I was nine years old.

"What kind of a relationship do you have with your mother?"

For some reason I stood up and angrily expressed exactly what was on my mind. She surprised me when she got up, walked over and placed both hands gently but firmly on my shoulders.

"Okay, that's enough," she said and walked back to her desk.

She sat down and stared at me as if waiting for a reaction.

"What's wrong? Did I say something inappropriate or something?" I asked.

"Your mother was overwhelmed," she replied calmly.

"Excuse me?" I said, starting to feel a little confused. "You don't want to hear what I have to say?"

She started to speak, but I didn't hear any of it as frustration suddenly took over.

"I'm really sorry, but I don't think I am going to get anywhere with this," I found myself saying.

I picked up my purse and simply walked out the door.

"I'm sure that was the shortest session she's ever had," I mumbled as I quickly walked to my car.

I was quite surprised at my own actions that day, and it took a while before the anger subsided. *Why was I so upset with her? Why did I have such a short fuse?* I knew Bruce was going to be disappointed with me, and I wasn't sure how I would explain.

By the time I reached home, I was feeling pretty bad.

"I don't think leaving was a good thing," he said after I explained how things went sideways. "Maybe you should make another appointment? She's a psychologist! She'd understand you were angry with your mother, not with her."

There's no way I will ever go back to that person, it won't work! I thought to myself.

"You're probably right," I said, "but let's wait a bit, let me get over my anger first."

I started to wonder if I was beyond help. Would talking to someone work after all? I decided to just let it all go and not think about it anymore.

As time went on, however, I found the challenge to control my triggers too difficult. The ups and downs on the mental and emotional levels continued, and so things remained pretty much the same. Stephen was still living at home but spent most of his time with his girlfriend who lived ten minutes away.

I had an unsavoury connection with a particular man who lived next door. My girlfriend Bobby jokingly described him as a relic of the past. Unfortunately, Stephen was drawn to him from an early age. He would fill the kids' minds with nonsense, and he encouraged bad behaviour. He snuck bottles of beer and cigarettes to Stephen when he was only ten years old and took pictures of him holding a bottle of beer and a cigarette.

I had many clashes with this guy, who also caused tension between Bruce and I, especially when he'd come into our yard. He took pleasure in the fact that his very presence was upsetting to me. I could never understand why Bruce turned a blind eye to this person's bad influence on Stephen. Why did he ignore this problem?

Thankfully, Robert was wise enough to turn away, and he always showed nothing but respect for us. Stephen considered me to be an over-protective mom. One time when I went next door to take Stephen home, this macho guy said to me "You know he's going to turn his back on you one of these days." Of course, Stephen absorbed all of this, and it made him even more obstinate whenever I had to step in.

I pointed out to Bruce that there had to be some kind of collaboration between us as parents in order for Stephen to get the right message, that he has to respect his parents. I was wasting my breath because nothing changed, and Stephen and I became more distant.

Another man lived across from the little lake near our house, and I ended up avoiding him as well. He was walking towards his truck that was parked in front of his garage. I was about to wave, but he hadn't seen me yet. Just then a cute little grey kitten appeared and started following him, meowing in a sort of pestering manner. When he reached to open the door of the truck, he almost stepped on it. He suddenly bent down, grabbed the innocent little kitten by the tail and flung it against the garage door! *Oh My God! That poor little kitten!* I turned and ran from the disgusting, cruel scene in shock and disbelief. The image haunted me for quite some time after that.

By the late 1980s, my relationship with Bruce was barely hanging by a thread. Even so, I hoped my mental condition would somehow improve and we might be able to salvage it. But I hadn't been receiving any treatment for my mental health issues, and I was not able to hold it together. By the end of 1987, we were divorced but still lived together even though we had signed legal papers. We cared for each other, but it was just not the same as in the beginning. I really had nowhere else to go, so life just went on as usual. I don't know of any couple who stayed living under the same roof after a divorce, and when I look back, I see how odd this arrangement was.

Chapter 18

I spent time in Ottawa with margiis Chris and Jane more often during the next few years, which helped a lot. All the while, though, I had this fantasy that I would eventually find a so-called soulmate. Even Bruce said he hoped I would eventually find what I was looking for.

One day I got a phone call from a police officer in Hamilton, a city at least eight hours' drive from where we lived. When the officer asked to speak with Robert, I thought there must be some kind of a mistake. *Why would the police have my son's phone number?* I thought. Robert, who was twenty years old at the time, was living and working in Montreal and had never been in trouble of any kind. I was dumbfounded!

"I'm sorry, but Robert is not here," I said.

When he inquired who Robert was and I told him he was my son, he explained that Lee, Robert's biological father whom we had not heard from since Robert was six months old, had been killed in a car crash in Hamilton. This phone number had been found in his wallet. It appeared that Lee had lost control of his van and veered off the highway and into the ditch. He died instantly. Lee had no living relatives to get in touch with, so they called this number.

Lee had a way of disconnecting from everyone once he decided to move on, so it looks like that's what happened when he disappeared a few years previous. I was grateful to have received the information from the Hamilton police, otherwise we would never have known.

Bruce and I were saddened by the news that Lee had ended up alone without any family, and that he had died in such a tragic way. Robert was too young to remember Lee, but I had a few photos of him holding Robert on his lap when he was six months old. I had always assumed Lee was living in Montreal, and I was disappointed when we hadn't heard from him. It's too bad things turned out that way, but I remind myself that everything is unfolding as it should throughout this universe, and that we are all being taken care of whether we are aware of it or not. I also believe that Lee is still with us in spirit. Robert is doing a great job raising his own little family as well.

I had some favourite spots to sit and meditate in the fields around our house, and I also had a particular trail I liked to walk along. I had never met anyone else while out on that trail over the years until one day when I was nearing the end of my long walk.

I was startled by what sounded like a chain rattling just behind me, but when I turned around, I couldn't see anything, just the clear path lined with trees. I heard a dog panting, and when I turned around again, I saw a neighbour with his German shepherd. When the dog stopped and stared at me for a second, I saw he was not attached to the chain leash the neighbour had in his hand. They were about thirty feet away when the dog suddenly started running towards me.

"STOP!" the man shouted.

But it did not yield. With no time to think or even react, I just froze in my tracks with my arms crossed over my chest and braced myself as the dog lunged forward. I could feel his front tooth break the skin on my arm.

"NO! NO!" the man yelled, catching him by the collar while forcing him to the ground.

I clutched my bleeding arm in a state of shock as he frantically tried to attach the chain leash to the collar. During that attack, my strength had instantly diminished, leaving me feeling weak and vulnerable. Holding my arm to my chest, I began to slowly walk away. I could hear him apologizing but didn't look back as I cautiously made my way across the field.

I drove straight to the clinic where I was given a shot for tetanus and my arm was put in a sling. When I returned home, Stephen was in the garage but wasn't at all concerned when he saw my injury. I said I had been bitten by a dog, but he continued with his head under the hood of the vehicle that he was working on without saying a word. It was little things like this that showed me how he couldn't care less about me, which hurt because I had always showed affection towards both kids equally.

My arm naturally healed with time, but the mental scars from the many traumas in my past didn't. They would influence my choices from there onward.

I wondered if I should stay there in the home we had built and loved dearly, or if I should find my future somewhere else. I felt the love just wasn't there anymore. I found myself constantly pondering the question, *Where do I go from here?* But I couldn't come up with an answer.

Meantime, I was in a different mindset when strolling the fields. I was constantly looking back to make sure it was safe, which broke the peace and contentment I had always experienced. I felt sad that I was losing my desire to even go there anymore. I often opted to walk along the road or go for a short bike ride instead.

By the end of the summer of 1997, I felt unwanted and had no connections with local margiis anymore. I woke one day with this lingering, awful and deep feeling of sadness I could not shake off. I couldn't even get into my yoga exercises or meditation I did regularly. I was not able to shed the feeling that I was worthless. I honestly felt that I was not worthy of love, and as crazy as it sounds, I even thought that God did not accept me anymore.

Wow, when I think about it now, I realize how pathetic and sad that was.

At the end of that day I was in the bathroom with a serious intention of slitting my wrists. I held a blade in my hand and tried to get up enough courage to just get it over with. But to my surprise, when I stepped into the tub and sat down, I suddenly began trembling as I took a deep breath and went to slice through the vein in my wrist. That's when an image of Robert suddenly flashed before me.

"NO! I can't let him find me like this! God help me!" I cried out as I came to my senses.

Stepping out of the tub, shaking from head to toe. I prayed as I ran to the phone; I needed to call someone—anyone! As I picked up the address book, my hands were shaking so badly it slipped and fell onto the counter face up. A telephone number jumped out at me, so I dialed it immediately.

Chris, one of the margiis from Ottawa, answered and was very surprised when I admitted what I had almost just done and explaining how volatile my situation had become. They had no idea Bruce and I were having problems. Chris suggested I come to Ottawa and stay with them over that weekend. He told me about a little village called Wakefield just thirty minutes north of Ottawa where some artists live and thought I might be interested in going there.

I could hardly get to sleep that night with this unexpected proposition swirling around in my head. There was this switch from hopelessness and despair to suddenly being optimistic. I knew I had better move on this right away, though, and the fear of changing my mind suddenly spurred me into action because I decided to leave as soon as possible. Interestingly enough, this happened to be on a Labour Day weekend—when most of the major changes in my life always seemed to occur.

I was determined to go through with this plan to find a place in Wakefield as they had recommended, and I was grateful that they cared enough to help out. Bruce was stunned when I told him what had taken place, but he also understood where I was coming from. Deep down, I knew he wished me well in my endeavour to find whatever I was looking for.

We had bought a new car, a Toyota Tercel, about a year before, so I was thankful when Bruce said I could take it when I left that weekend. I said my goodbyes and asked the Supreme for guidance as I headed for the highway. I truly believed that this was meant to be—that, yes, I was doing the right thing at the right time. I felt it in my soul.

Chapter 19

I stopped along the way to rest as I normally did on my trips to Ottawa, and when I finally arrived, I was full of hope. Even though I knew being in my mid-fifties and taking on this change would not be easy, I took the plunge anyway.

The margii family was receptive and willing to get me started, so I was shown the route to Wakefield and left early the next morning. The thirty-minute drive ended at the bottom of a hill in the village where the road came to a T-intersection at the water's edge. At the stop sign, I gazed out at the tranquil scene in front of me, so calm and inviting, with the bright sun sparkling on the lake. As I sat there for a moment wondering which way to turn, the shrill sound of a loon pierced the silence. Oh how beautiful!

Someone was sitting on the deck of the restaurant at the intersection, so I rolled the window down and asked, "Which way to the General Store?" He pointed to the left, so I slowly drove along what was obviously the main street until I came to the General Store.

Inside on their bulletin board I found a notice that said "House to share." It was owned by a young professional woman named Lora who worked for the government in Ottawa. I took her phone number and headed right back to Ottawa. After a short chat over the phone, she gave me her address and asked if I could come to her place that evening around seven o'clock. I had been at her house only a few minutes when she told me, yes, I could share the house with her. I went directly to bed when I got back to Ottawa because I was beginning to have pain in my head, which was normal for me when under stress. Actually it had been slowly mounting from the moment I woke up that morning.

The next morning I went to apply for government assistance as Chris had suggested, but never having done anything like this before I found the whole procedure to be quite stressful. I then headed up to Wakefield with the documents in hand that I was told had to be signed by a doctor in order to have the medical attention I needed.

As I drove along the main street, I was relieved to see there was a chiropractor near the family clinic in Wakefield where I would have the papers signed by a physician. I entered his office and sat down at his desk feeling quite timid and unsure of myself. He looked at me with a friendly smile and said, "So what is your problem?" I handed him the papers and explained the situation. He signed the papers, and as I wrote his name in my little address book, *Dr. Folkerson*, he noticed my hand was shaking.

"Okay, first thing I think we'll do is get you an appointment with a psychotherapist," he said. "And if you wish, you can see her here at the Wakefield Memorial Hospital on a regular basis. Her name is Louise Roy. Hum, I see a note here that says you have just separated from your husband after twenty seven years," he said with empathy.

I was so thankful that he didn't question me or create any unnecessary obstacles.

"Yes, I did," I said. "Thank you for signing the papers. I see there's a chiropractor near here. Do you think there's any chance I'd get to see someone there today?"

"I'll try to arrange that for you while you're here; let me give them a call."

By the time I left his office I was almost numb from the pain, but I was amazed at how everything was actually working out in my favour. It was almost too good to be true. I was able to go directly from the clinic straight to the chiropractor. After my treatment, I was tired and aching all over, and I just wanted to get back to Ottawa. But first I stopped by the General

Store to grab something to eat—I was so hungry. I spotted the tomatoes as I walked in and picked up one large ripe one, then I grabbed a package of burger buns along with a drink. From there, I went outside and sat down at the water's edge. I remember biting into the tomato as if it were an apple, and how incredibly delicious it was. Even the plain bun tasted better than usual, probably because I was famished. Feeling rather sleepy, I crawled into the back seat of my car and dozed off before heading back to Ottawa.

The next morning, I left the margii's house for the thirty-minute drive to Lora's place with great anticipation for what laid ahead. Her home was a lovely large white cottage next to a golf course with only a few neighbours close by. She was friendly enough but didn't say much, which was fine with me. Actually, I appreciated the privacy and was able to begin my much-needed healing process shortly after I arrived.

A simple thing like going out for short walks with her little dog was the highlight of each day. When Chris came by a few weeks later to see how I was doing, I told him I felt ready to move forward even though it seemed as if I had a mountain in front of me yet to climb. I figured I could do it if I stuck to my spiritual practices, attended regular therapy sessions and received chiropractic treatments.

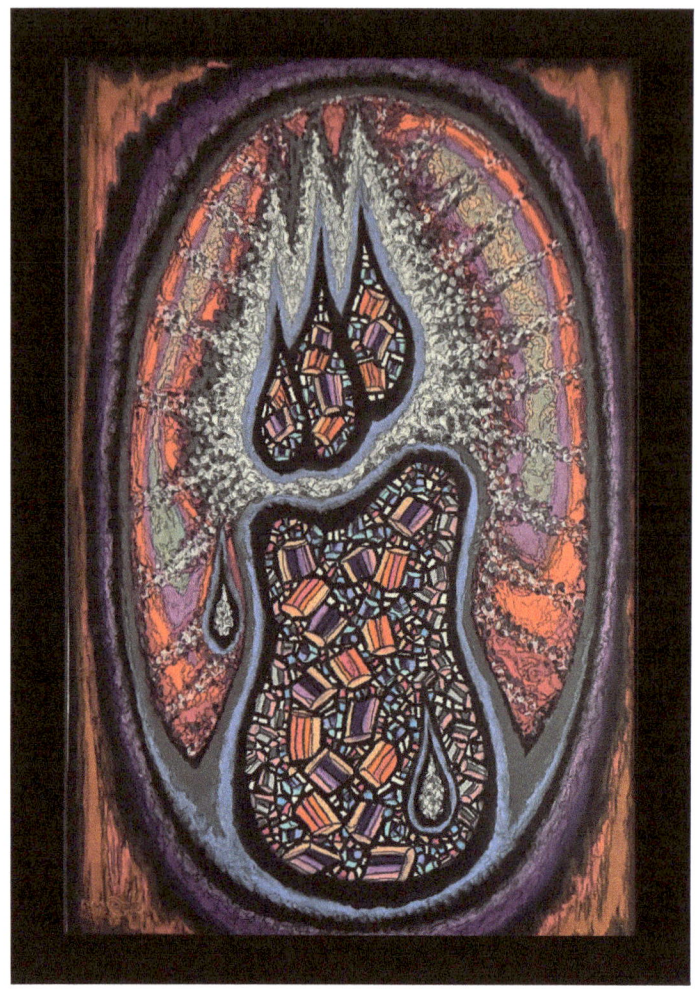

HOPE IN THE NIGHT
The 3 flames represent struggle on 3 levels -
physical, mental and spiritual

I even held onto my belief that I might eventually find my so-called soulmate one day. This would be an ideal situation. Even though I was fifty-five years old, I was a young fifty-five, if I do say so myself, and I was determined to achieve my goal. From the time I arrived on that Labour Day weekend through to the middle of November, I became stronger on all levels.

There were moments when I shed some tears but never when Lora was at home; a short bout and it was over with. I always knew it would pass because I was able to immediately replace a negative thought with a positive one. I reminded myself to be grateful for what I had instead of feeling sad for what I didn't. It actually worked, but it took some effort.

One day without any warning whatsoever, everything suddenly turned upside down. I had made some vegetarian burgers, put a batch in the freezer and then gone upstairs to my room to meditate and rest as usual. I always got my own groceries and did my own cooking, of course, which I preferred to do during the week while Lora was at work in Ottawa. There I was in my room at the end of what seemed like a reasonably good day, when I opened a box containing some family photos of Robert, Stephen, Bruce and myself. It was the first time I'd looked at them since I had arrived two and a half months before. My happiness to look at them gradually changed to sadness, and I began to reflect on the all-encompassing picture of my life, including the traumas of the twenty-seven years I spent with Bruce.

A tear trickled down my cheek, so I put the pictures away and reminded myself to focus on positive thoughts only. I intended to bounce back as I usually did, but it didn't work this time. I began sobbing quietly into my pillow. I shouldn't have looked at the pictures, they only brought on feelings of disconnect and isolation. Wanting to suppress emotions that were pulling me down, I tried to console myself with, *Others have gone through much more in their lives and managed to move on, I can too!* But a loud knock on my bedroom door jolted me out of my pity party.

"Anna Maria?"

Oh no! Lora's back! Get a grip on yourself, you can't let her see you in this condition!

"Can I come in?" she asked.

I braced myself, forcing a smile as I opened the door.

"Were you crying? I thought I could hear you crying?" she said with a slight frown.

"No, I'm okay."

She could see I was trying to hide the tears, and it was clear she was not about to let it go so easily. Stepping into the room, she stood in front of me and stared into my eyes with this intense look on her face.

"I heard you crying. So what's wrong? Did something happen while I was gone?"

The only thing that Lora knew was what I had told her in that short interview: that I had left my husband after twenty seven-years and was staying with the margii family in Ottawa while looking for a place to live in Wakefield. Because of the stigma associated with mental illness, I was afraid she might turn me away, so I thought it would be better to not say anything about it. I was caught up in the moment that day, and I felt obliged to answer her persistent questioning. It was an awkward moment for both of us.

"I don't mean to pry, but what happened?"

"I was having a difficult time trying to move on from the past," I replied.

"Was your husband abusive?" she asked.

"No, no, nothing like that." I didn't know what to say next. "But I will be more careful not to disturb you from now on."

"I'm curious, why did you leave after twenty-seven years?"

"Well … um, actually I decided I should leave when I began to have suicidal thoughts …"

"You WHAT?"

She backed away with a look of fear on her face, then in an angry tone, she said, "Well, just don't do anything in MY house!"

She turned and stomped out the door.

I stood there staring in disbelief as she disappeared downstairs and out the front door in a huff. Seconds later, she drove off in her jeep. I was beyond shocked. I collapsed on the bed and burst into tears.

"No—NOOO! I shouldn't have told her!"

The reality of what happened shook me to the core. I'd have to find another place and face the possibility of yet another rejection. It was just too much. I lost it completely. I slid to my knees on the floor and leaned over the edge of the bed, hands folded in prayer.

"GOD!" I cried out. "I thought you were taking care of me! So why? WHY is this happening?"

Two words kept repeating in my mind: *Call Louise! Call Louise!* She had been my therapist for the previous two and a half months, so I reached for the phone and dialled her number (which I knew off by heart). When she answered I was sobbing so hard she couldn't understand what I was saying.

"It's Anna Maria!" I finally blurted out.

"Okay," she said calmly. "Come directly to the emergency. I will be waiting for you at the entrance."

Everything was a blur as I rushed down and jumped into my car, still sobbing uncontrollably and feeling totally abandoned. I was afraid for what might happen when Lora returned. I was truly devastated. With no hope on the horizon, I grappled with thoughts of suicide as I sped along the highway, blinded by tears.

I'll just slam into the next pole! Too late! The next one then!

Straining to see more clearly, I suddenly spotted a road sign on my left that read "Burnside." It's where I had to turn off to get to the Wakefield Memorial Hospital, so I pumped the brakes and made a sharp turn left. It dawned on me how insane this was and just how close I had come to taking my own life. Again! With that sobering thought in mind, I clung onto the words Louise said over the phone: "I'll be waiting for you." Sure enough, she was there standing at the door waiting for me.

"Thank God," I whispered as I pulled into a parking spot close to the entrance.

She greeted me with a warm smile, a moment I shall never forget. I felt as if I had just been rescued by an angel.

"Good, you've calmed down. Let's get you inside where we can talk."

I followed her into her office and, feeling emotionally safe, I was able to clarify my hysterical gibberish from the phone. I knew she understood my plight, so I was able to get my bearings and listen to her.

"Louise, there are no words to express how grateful I am that you were there for me when I called. Honestly, I don't think I would have made it this far without your help," I said. "You have been there for me right from the beginning when I came to Wakefield two and a half months ago. Leaving home at that time I never would have imagined running into a situation such as this—never! But now that I've made it this far, I want to keep moving forward. I don't want to dwell on the past, it will only slow me down. I realize I must find another place to live, so maybe I should check out the *Wakefield News* to see if there's a room I could rent. Lora's house can't be the only place around. What do you think?"

"We can certainly discuss this further now that you're here," she said. "What was on your mind just before you made that call? I think you should stay here overnight, Anna Maria, so Dr. Folkerson and I can come by to see you in the morning. We'll give you a sedative to help get you through the night, okay?"

"Yes, thank you."

The next morning I awoke to the sound of voices speaking in a low, hushed tone. When I opened my eyes, I was a bit groggy but could see the back of someone whom I figured was a nurse. She was having a conversation with someone in the hallway. Then she stepped aside as if allowing that person to come into the room. My eyes popped wide open when I saw it was Lora! She quickly but cautiously approached me with an envelope.

"Sorry, but I am not going to be your caretaker," she said in a matter-of-fact tone.

As she walked away, I thought, *What's this?* I opened the envelope to find a typed letter stating she and I had come to an agreement that I was no longer sharing the house as of yesterday. I was surprised, to say the least, since we'd never had any kind of agreement. In fact, I was stunned and totally confused when she left.

Fortunately, because I was now in a safe place, that letter and the manner in which she approached me didn't set me back. It actually showed me how much strength I had now that I was receiving proper medical attention and was surrounded by people who cared about what happened to me. So I put the letter aside, vowing not to let incidences such as this get in my way.

Just then Dr. Folkerson and Louise came into the room. I didn't mention that Lora dropped by with the letter.

"How are you doing this morning?" Louise wanted to know.

I felt like giving them both a hug for being earth angels.

"You have no idea what you have done for me," I said.

"Well, we do our best to accommodate everyone, and we're glad to see you're doing better this morning," said Louise. "So I have some news for you. We think it's best that you remain here in the hospital for the next two weeks while we find a place for you to stay in the Wakefield area."

It was as if a weight had been lifted off my shoulders.

"I don't know what to say, I am so very grateful."

"So there is nothing to worry about," Dr. Folkerson said.

When they left, a surge of hope welled up inside. *I will make it out there after all; life I will be worth living despite the challenges waiting for me,* I thought. When I left home on that Labour Day weekend in September, I knew it wouldn't be easy, but at least I had enough support to help carry me through. With this in mind, I turned over and fell into a deep sleep, knowing that healing had already begun.

Chapter 20

Because I was there in the hospital, I was able to attend therapy sessions with Louise more often. When the two weeks were up, she informed me that she had been in touch with a woman whose name also happened to be Louise. She was the founder of a group home called Maison Le Ricochet (meaning to bounce back into society). She had bought a motel a few years ago to convert into a residence for people who were in situations like mine.

"Louise Beauchemin also works in this group home where you will be living, Louise my therapist said. It's in Masham, only ten minutes away from the hospital. Since I go over on a regular basis, we will be able to continue with our therapy sessions from there, no problem."

It was the middle of December 1997, and I was on the move again.

A tall, nice looking gentleman who was probably in his forties came to pick me up. His name was Carol. I understood he was in charge when Louise Beauchemin was not there.

"Someone will come to drive your car over to Le Ricochet, so you can leave your keys with me," he said.

I handed them over as we walked to his van that was waiting in front of the entrance. After a rather short drive, we turned into the driveway of a well-kept one-storey brick building. You would think it was a private home with the trimmed cedar hedge across the front and large wooden swing near the front door. The whole place was dusted in snow. The building extended way back onto the property, which were obviously the rooms when it had been a motel.

Entering through the front door, the open concept of the kitchen and dining room on my left was bright and welcoming. On the right side, the living room had a fire burning in the fireplace with chopped wood sitting on a grate next to it. *How cozy,* I thought, but I didn't see anyone yet.

Carol led me to a conference room that had chairs and a long table; there was a small sitting room across from it. Just then a female voice called, "Carol? Is that you?" We stepped down into the long hallway and saw whom I figured was Louise sitting behind her desk.

"Thank you, Carol," she said with a big smile as she stood up to greet us.

She was probably in her mid-forties and had black hair done in a modern style to go with her lovely outfit.

"Hello, Anna Maria, and welcome!" she said with such strong positive energy I couldn't help but connect with her immediately. "So we'll put you in the room next to my office here, and your car will be parked right there in front of your window."

"This is much more than I expected, thank you so much Louise."

She then briefed me on the day's schedule.

"Carol will be here till four o'clock, that's when someone else will come in and take over until midnight. Another worker will do the shift from midnight to eight in the morning, so someone is here twenty-four hours a day. If you need anything or just want to talk, don't hesitate. Louise Roy will see you every two weeks here as well."

"I'm leaving now. I have a long list of groceries as usual," Carol said. "If there's anything you need, I'll add it now."

"No thank you, I will be happy with whatever they have. One thing I won't have, though, is meat; I am a vegetarian," I said.

Louise went back to her work and I went to my room, closed the door and just laid there for a few minutes. This was a lot to take in. I had a flashback of my struggles to find proper care and attention, and couldn't help but see how this situation I'd stepped into was nothing short of a miracle. This realization of how the Supreme was always guiding me inspired me to get up and spend the next hour in deep meditation.

At supper time that evening, I met another caregiver, Cheryl, a caring woman around Carol's age with big, beautiful blue eyes and blond hair. We clicked immediately. She told me about Lac Philippe in Gatineau Park, which was only a two-minute drive from the residence. I could swim there in the summer and walk on the paths along the lake, which would help a lot in the healing process. I could hardly believe it.

Finally, I met the other eight people who were living there as we sat for supper at the long table, but I did not feel open to being friendly with anyone just yet. I only connected with Cheryl and Carol. I thanked them for making me feel so welcome, and I went straight to my room after dinner.

That night I had a true revelation. In my mind, I saw the image of a small plaque of the poem *Footprints* I used to have on my fridge at home. There was an indentation of a set of footprints in the sand along with these words:

FOOTPRINTS
"My precious child,
I never left you during your time of trial.
Where you see only one set of FOOTPRINTS,
It was then that I carried you."

The words struck a cord in my brain and it dawned on me that, I had definitely been guided from the time I left home on that Labour Day weekend to when I was finally brought to Le Maison Ricochet in Masham.

I was able to comprehend this on the spiritual level, so I continued to move forward remembering that I was not alone. As our guru used to say, "You are never alone or helpless; the force that guides the stars, guides you too." I now understood that what I thought was the worst thing that could have happened (being evicted) was actually the best thing after all. By having to leave Lora's place as I did, I gained immediate access to the care I so desperately needed for my mental health. It was crystal clear that the right connections were definitely being made at the right time. This revelation gave me the strength I needed to get past the inevitable obstacles as I began the next chapter in my life.

Since I always had a problem with interpersonal relationships, I was concerned about how vulnerable I was while living in such close proximity with the others who were going through difficult times as well. I didn't know how it might affect me emotionally. At least I had my therapist Louise's unwavering support. I had an appointment with her in a few days, so I tried not to worry about it.

When I was living with Lora, I wanted to be sure I was strong enough mentally before getting in touch with Bruce and Robert. My intention was to let them know what was happening with me as soon as I felt stable and more in control of my emotions. I wanted to give them good news about how well I was doing. I was almost at that point when the unexpected eviction happened, causing me to suddenly spiral downwards. I thought I should put off contacting them once again as I didn't want them to know I had been evicted. Not yet anyway.

When Christmas arrived, I was amazed that Louise Beauchemin had organized a wonderful Christmas party with catered food, great music and gifts for everyone. Carol was Santa Claus, and we all thoroughly enjoyed sharing in the festive season that year. I still have a beautiful white robe with gold trim that she gave me as a Christmas present. It is a reminder of her generosity and support while I was there.

I was at Le Ricochet about three weeks when I finally felt ready to connect with Bruce and Robert again. They were happy for me when I told them about the incredible care and attention I was getting in Masham. I told them about Lora and being evicted, which led to my hospital stay just before I ended up at Le Ricochet. I knew they cared about what happened to me, and I didn't want either of them to worry about how I was making out on my own. They understood that I knew my faith would guide me to the right place at the right time, so they were relieved to hear that's exactly what happened during those two and a half months when they didn't hear from me.

There was more to Le Ricochet than what was visible upon arrival. They had a place a short drive away from the residence where we could do ceramics, woodwork, art, stained glass, etc. Plus, there was a lovely boutique just a few minutes' walk away where Le Ricochet sold second-hand clothing that was like new. Those who were well enough and interested in working there were more than welcome to do so. It helped them to have more confidence in themselves and to become more independent.

Some of the residents were able to return home to their families, but once in a while someone came back for a short stay if they ran into problems or had been prescribed a change in medication. The support they needed was always there. There was a two-year limit for anyone to stay, but most did not stay that long because they moved on and functioned on their own.

I began to wake up during the night quite often, something I never experienced before. When I couldn't get back to sleep, I'd sit and meditate, but I was unable to concentrate on my mantra, so that didn't work. I'd look for something in the fridge to comfort me, which helped.

Sometimes when sitting in meditation in the middle of the night, my mind would simply go blank and I'd feel tears running down my face. This was bizarre since there were no images in my mind, so I couldn't for the life of me figure out why I was crying. Normally a person would have some idea at least of why they were crying, but I didn't. So instead of reaching for something to snack on, which I knew was becoming a habit and bothered me quite a bit, I just sat quietly and let the tears flow. I would get back into bed when it stopped.

This continued for at least two months, so therapist Louise and I were concerned. Aside from my emotional eating problem that had started recently, we couldn't figure out where all these tears were coming from. We decided to give it some time and see if it would just stop on its own, which, thankfully, it did.

I struggled to deal with some bad connections at Le Ricochet at times, and I wondered how I'd manage if I was triggered. But according to therapist Louise, I was doing pretty well compared to when I first arrived. Even so, I still had a lot of work to do regarding my "approach," as she put it, when dealing with other residents, including the caregivers. I was terribly worried about this.

I got along well with Carol and Cheryl. Then there was Julie, a sweet new caregiver in her late twenties whom I liked very much. There was also the mayor's wife, Clair, who was the nurturing type. They all took courses in mental health while working there and were clearly capable when handling the residents. Then there was this new guy who had been hired for the shift from four o'clock to midnight. I felt like he did not like me at all, and he often ignored me when I needed attention.

When I discovered he had worked as a prison guard in the past, it put me on alert. His manner was not gentle and he didn't care for us as the other workers did, so I soon became apprehensive about approaching him when I needed something. So I didn't say anything because I felt I might get blamed if there was a problem.

A huge ice storm that cut the electricity off to a large area in the province of Quebec, including Le Ricochet, hit. Thankfully, they were equipped with a reliable generator, so it wasn't an issue. I heard that a section of Montreal where Robert lived was also hit, so I immediately went to the phone in the kitchen to call him using my calling card. I had trouble connecting properly. This particular caregiver happened to be sitting in the living room watching TV, and he could see how frustrated I was getting, but he didn't blink an eye when he saw I was in need of some assistance. I finally slammed the receiver down in frustration when I couldn't connect.

"What are you doing?" he asked in a demanding tone like I was in trouble.

"I can't reach my son in Montreal—I want to know if he's okay!" I said on the verge of tears.

My brain is not able to think at times. I simply needed his assistance, but he completely ignored me, took his paperwork and sat down at the dining room table.

"I want to talk to my son!" I said again.

"Well, I can't do anything about that!" he said flatly.

I felt hurt and was about to run to my room, but instead, I sat down and just stared at him with daggers in my eyes. He clearly didn't get it, it just went over his head. There was a small piece of paper on the table that he had just rolled up and threw to the side with impatience, as if I was disturbing him. I felt anger rise up inside, reached for the paper and tore small bits off. I rolled them into tight, tiny balls, and when I saw he was determined to get rid of me, I flicked one his way.

"You're being rude!" he said angrily.

"And you're IGNORING ME!" I shot back.

He continued writing, so I got up and left, knowing he was not about to help in any way. I tossed and turned that night, wondering if Robert was all right while being anxious and afraid of what tomorrow might bring.

The next morning when I mentioned it to Louise, she asked Clair (who was on duty) to help me get in touch with Robert. I was relieved to hear he had not been affected by the ice storm after all.

There were similar incidents with this new caregiver, and it caused a lot of anxiety for me whenever he came into work. He made the residents form a line in order to receive their medication, for instance, which the other caregivers didn't do. Mine happened to be hormone pills, so I didn't think

I should have to get in line for that. The other caregivers gave the residents their medication at meal times when they came to the table, so when I was preparing my own dinner and he called my name to come for the pills, I said politely, "Would you mind just leaving them there on my plate?"

"No—come here," he said, making me feel like I was some kind of an inmate in a prison.

This may not sound like something to be disturbed about, but his uncaring attitude really struck a nerve with me. Especially when I saw his intention was to be more in control of everyone, which I resented. I even began to suspect he wanted to get rid of me, but I vowed that if it came down to him or me staying, I definitely was not going to be the one to have to go.

The tension escalated to the point where everyone at the table was aware of the friction between us. Frustrated and angry, I left the food I was preparing there on the cupboard and walked out the door. It didn't do much good because I only became more fearful of being kicked out as I walked back to the residence. As I came back in, he approached me with such an authoritarian manner, that it instantly threw me into a defensive mode.

"You're not having me put out!" I said as I shoved him aside and walked to my room.

I was seething with anger, but I was more afraid of what awaited me when Louise read his report. So I was awake most of the night.

The next morning, I went for my walk as usual after meditating and doing yoga, and who was coming up our street but Louise Beauchemin. She blew the horn and gave a big wave. *I don't know how happy she'll be when she finds out about last night,* I thought. I really did want to co-operate with the workers and adapt accordingly, but this particular caregiver wasn't even up to par in my estimation. My emotional needs were quite simple, actually, once you knew what they were. But he wasn't interested in knowing. In my opinion he was driven by a need to be in total control, which would never work with someone like me. There was a heavy cloud looming, and I had no idea what to do to make it go away.

Sure enough, when Louise read his report, she called me into the conference room where she held her regular meetings.

"We have a problem," she said in a serious tone.

Oh no, I thought, *she's about to throw me out!*

She asked me about the night before, and when I explained my side and how he affected me in such a negative way, she said, "I will talk to him when he comes in this evening. I want to see if he is lacking."

With that, she gently dismissed me. I didn't know what to think or how to react, but I knew I had to be prepared for the worst while hoping for the best. It reminded me of the experiences I'd had in the past. I was really uptight while waiting for her assessment, and I anticipated problems when this worker came in at four o'clock for his evening shift. I also had bouts of crying like I used to have when I was at Lora's place. The stress was really getting to me.

However, when I came up to the dining table for supper at five o'clock, I did not see the male caregiver. Cheryl was serving the food and being her sweet self, as usual. She wanted to know if I was going to make my own meal or if I wanted what the others were having. I was not in the cooking mood, so I opted to have the same as the others but without the meat. I couldn't keep quiet any longer, so I asked if he was coming in to work or not.

"Oh, Louise told me she's giving him a two-week vacation," Cheryl replied.

Those words were like music to my ears. I felt my entire body let go of the tension I was holding with a huge sigh of relief.

"Thank God," I said, grateful to be able to have a normal evening for a change.

I was glad it turned out to be Cheryl taking his place.

By March, I was looking forward to the snow melting so I could drive over to Lac Phillipe in Gatineau Park. There were cross-country skiing and snowshoeing trails, but I wasn't interested. I kept myself busy with my artwork, which Louise thought was a great way to spend my time while going through my much-needed healing period. She recognized how much effort I had put into staying balanced on all levels.

I had gotten myself into a regular routine that was quite different from the others. I kept up with my meditation and exercises along with my artwork while I was there instead of going to the workshops that kept people occupied. But I eventually went to one where I made a nice stained-glass vase which I have in my living room to this day.

In the weeks that followed, I got in touch with Bruce and Robert again but hadn't had any connection with Anita yet. I heard she was doing okay in her marriage with George, the long-distance truck driver. It was great to see Robert again when he came to the residence and brought four or five pieces of my framed art from home that I asked for along with a particular type of paper I needed to do my work. So I was able to get back into creating again. I also put my framed work up on the walls in my little apartment to help inspire me to continue.

Louise decided it was time for me to move from my room next to her office to one of the two little apartments at the end of the hall. It had a fridge, stove, sink and shower. I began to cook my own meals instead of going to the dining room with everyone else, and I bought my own groceries since I had my own car.

Before Louise left for her March break, she bought a couple of cans of yellow paint and asked if I'd like to paint my little one-room apartment while she was gone.

"I'll come back and see what you did with it," she said.

I was so afraid I'd make a mess of it, but I did my best. I cried off and on because I was so anxious about her reaction when she got back, but she thought it was okay, so I was relieved. To my surprise, she called me into the conference room shortly afterwards and told me she wanted to redo the kitchen and dining room floors.

"We're going to put new tiles down and we'd like you to help choose the colours," she said.

She realized just how insecure I was when I hesitated and said "Ummm … I don't think so."

I wanted to please her but was too scared I'd make the wrong choice. I was slightly embarrassed, so I excused myself. I was okay with my art because I just had to please myself, so I was satisfied with the colours I'd choose. But this was something else, and I wasn't sure if I would do it correctly.

Not only were they renovating the existing building, but they also planned to expand and accommodate the clothing store and workshops, making it much larger with more offices for the staff. They also wanted to add another large conference room and kitchen. It was going to be state of the art, as Louise would say. It turned out to be a beautiful complex. The residents even made some lovely large wooden picnic tables and swings that held four people.

Occasionally when I came back from my walk in the morning, I'd find an envelope at my door with a beautiful card from Louis Beauchemin inside. She encouraged me to stay strong, and she praised my artwork and my efforts to move forward despite the obstacles in my path. She totally understood my struggles with my mental condition. Actually, she had a son who was about twelve years old who also had some mental health issues.

A few people in the community had resisted having this complex in the neighbourhood in the beginning. But with her extraordinary tenacity, she managed to convince them that this would be a great place to help those who were in need of such a place. I admired her very much.

I was doing better than ever mainly because the connections I had were exactly what I needed to stay on track. I began to wonder whether that caregiver I had a difficult time with would be back. Would I be able to stay balanced and strong enough when faced with him again? It bothered me to the extent that I went to Louise's office and asked her when he'd be back.

"No, don't worry, Anna Maria, he will not be coming back to work here. We have seen you are doing just fine when relating to the other caregivers. By the way, we would like you to display one of your paintings during a conference we are organizing."

I was surprised to hear this, and it did give me a boost in confidence. But mostly I was grateful for her understanding of how difficult it was for me to connect emotionally with others. In turn, I decided to give some of my time to Le Ricochet by helping out somehow.

"What do you think of me volunteering to work in the clothing store by helping to sort out the clothes coming in for donation?" I asked Louise Roy at my next appointment. "I saw a couple of the residents doing that while I was there."

"Are you happy now?" she asked.

I was taken aback, and said, "Yes, especially since I don't have to deal with that male caregiver anymore, thanks to Louise Beauchemin."

"Good. You will definitely need more time for healing though," she said. "So I don't think you should work in the store. Put your time and energy into your artwork and staying healthy. You seem to be happy now ... so let's keep it that way."

I thought about what she said and realized she was right. She once told me that sometimes when we're in the process of healing we mistakenly think we are better because we happen to feel better. But in fact we need to take more time to recover. I figured this must be true in my case, so I continued to rely more on her for advice and direction. I really don't know how I would have progressed without her constant support. I called her my earth angel. It's an affectionate name I used for those people who helped me as I struggled through so many different situations.

Bruce and I began writing short letters back and forth, and when the snow disappeared, he came over to see for himself how I was doing. I was happy to see him again, and we even considered the possibility of getting back together in the not-too-distant future. But to my dismay, Louise had some doubts when I mentioned this to her. She didn't actually come out and say it, but I saw from her frown while jotting a note.

"Hum, are you sure this is a good idea, Anna Maria?" she asked.

I was careful not to jump too quickly, which I had a tendency to do in the past.

When I went over to Lac Philippe for the first time, I explored the area close to the lake where I had parked and instantly felt as if I were in a magical place. I found a beautiful spot under a huge pine tree a few feet from the beach and sat down. I felt my entire nervous system become calm, and after about an hour of deep meditation, I walked along the path that ran along the edge of the lake. A couple of canoes, a few kayaks and a small sailboat could be seen out on the water. It was so quiet, only the chirping of the birds with the occasional call of a loon could be heard. I noticed a sign showing no motorboats were allowed, making it a perfect place to find peace and quiet. I knew then and there that this was definitely what my creator had in store for me. This was the place where I was meant to be during that summer of 1998, and I could not have been more grateful. Lac Philippe became the place I could go to contemplate and seek peace of mind, especially on those days when I really needed to be alone.

I believe my faith played a big part in helping me feel secure and protected while I was there. Having always kept my connection with my soul-self through the regular spiritual practices, I just knew deep down that there would always be some way to get past the roadblocks on this difficult journey through life. I did not know how long I would be living at the residence, so I just took it one day at a time as planned.

Chapter 21

Every once in a while, I'd get my French tapes out that I brought from home and practice with the caregivers. It took some time before I attempted to actually speak to anyone in the grocery stores or the bank, for example, which reminded me of when I lived with Bruce over the past twenty-seven years. From the very beginning, when he saw I couldn't communicate with the French-speaking people properly, I'd wait in the car instead of going into the bank or even the grocery store sometimes. However, because I kept myself disconnected from everyone, including my neighbours, I slowly but surely began to feel the effects.

When I look back now, I see how much of a stumbling block that was for me to stay disconnected like that. Unfortunately, I didn't even recognize it as an impediment. But now, being in another place and time, I had to face the fact I would have to contend with this ongoing struggle within. That it was not good for me to continue to distance myself from people like that.

This was in the fall of 1998, and I still had this urge to drive back to Saint-Jean-de-Matha to see the house we had built and where we'd raised Robert and Stephen. But when I mentioned it to him in a letter, he wrote back that he had planned on coming to Le Ricochet soon to put up a garage-like tent he'd bought to protect my car during the winter snowstorms.

About a week later, he and Stephen showed up and erected the garage in the back of the residence close to my apartment. I made vegetarian burgers, home-made vegetable soup and muffins for them while they were busy outside, expecting the three of us would have lunch together. But Stephen declined, wanting to leave as soon as they finished putting the garage up. I was disappointed that he was still very distant and did not want to have anything to do with me. It reminded me of how our relationship was before I had left home. Regardless, I was thankful to both of them for giving of their time and energy. I never took anything for granted, which Bruce knew. He remained supportive and kind while I was at the residence and afterwards as well.

The leaves were nearing their peak of changing colours when I decided to go back to gather up anything—winter clothes and personal items—I'd forgotten to take with me when I'd left a year before. This was a good time, I thought, to see what it would be like should we actually get back together again. I sensed Bruce had concerns regarding my triggers, and even though I hadn't had any lately, we just didn't know what to expect in the coming weeks or months.

He was aware that Louise Roy thought I needed more time to heal before making any decisions regarding our relationship. I understood she was being objective and her primary concern was to keep me from stepping back into a situation that would not be conducive to my mental and emotional well-being. I did want to adhere to her cautionary advice, but I was pulled by my desire to go back. I wondered how I would feel after a year of separation. I was certain when I left home that I would not return, so I did not expect I would ever reconsider.

Anyway, there I was on my way back home to Saint-Jean-de-Matha with this big question mark in my mind about whether or not I was doing the right thing. I was thinking that with this visit we'd have a chance to see if there was any change for the better when it came to my mental condition. I was hoping we'd be able to pick up the pieces, so to speak, and make things work out somehow.

As I reached that rest area close to home where I barely escaped with my life, I had a flashback which made me cringe. I thought about the many obstacles I'd managed to kick aside as I made my way in life, and I vowed to continue my search for lasting happiness in whatever time I had left on this earth. If it wasn't with Bruce, then I had to seek out my soulmate. But I really wanted Bruce and I to make an effort first.

When I got back, we were more interested in how we would contend with our relationship on a day-to-day basis rather than becoming intimate with one another. We knew only too well how easily things could get out of hand should I suffer a trigger; it could ruin our chance of making any progress. We were actually more polite with one another than anything else when I arrived. Bruce slept on the couch in the living room while I was in the bedroom with our two cats. They purred as if they were happy I was back, but I tossed and turned with the same pain in my head that always accompanied any long drives. I got up and took a couple of painkillers, which finally helped put me to sleep.

It was probably three o'clock in the morning when I woke up to the moon shining through the window directly onto my face. I got up to pull the blind down and got back into bed expecting to fall back to sleep, but for some reason I wasn't able to. Instead, my mind rehashed many things that had taken place before I decided to finally leave a year before. So when I began to have that old feeling of needing to talk as I used to, I was afraid. Whenever I reached out to connect, I almost always ended up with a feeling of rejection, causing terrible triggers. I definitely did not want to go there ever again!

I wanted to let go of this need to talk that was taking hold in my mind, so I decided to go outside. Since there was a full moon, I could see clearly enough to take a little stroll around the yard. The pine and spruce trees we had planted all along the cedar fence when we built the house were now so tall that they cast long shadows across the yard. I gazed up at the silent stars to find the big dipper along with other formations that I used to look for when I'd sit outside on nights like this.

It was a bit chilly, so I went inside to put my housecoat on before heading back out into the yard. The air was so fresh and clean, as always, and the silence was so peaceful. As I made my way along the cedar fence in the backyard, I spotted the three little white signs that were nailed to the fence.

Each was about four by eight inches and had the names of our pets written on them. Our two little dogs, Tootsie and Tiny, along with our cat Mitsu were buried there, each in their own space and time. We treated them like members of the family.

I remembered how they used to accompany me on Monday mornings when I'd hang the clothes out to dry from the back step on those bright sunny days. Actually, I made a picture of just that years later. It shows a young mother reaching up to take the sheets off the line, and I titled it *Wind and Sun Dried*. It expressed that fresh, clean smell and feel of the clothes just after they had been blowing in the wind for a couple of hours. I totally appreciated my automatic washer and dryer, of course, and couldn't imagine having to do without them. I knew first-hand what drudgery it was when I started out with an old-fashioned wringer as a young mother years ago in New Waterford.

I was feeling pretty sentimental as I stood there remembering the days we had spent together as a family. We actually did share some happy times. "It wasn't all bad," as Bruce said to me a while back. I seemed to dwell on the difficult times and the triggers, but they were not an everyday occurrence. Being fortunate enough to find Le Ricochet in Masham and begun to heal, I assumed it would be just a matter of time before I was able to live a more normal life and not have to deal with triggers. I figured when I knew more, I'd be able to prevent them. At least I now had this hope to cling to.

But I began to have conflicting emotions as I tried to get past tonight's unexpected need to talk things out. I came back into the house and sat on the edge of the bed wondering whether or not I should wake Bruce, but I decided I'd better hold off until the morning. I did not want to disturb him even though it was the weekend and he didn't have to get up early in the morning. He always kept a fire going in the wood stove in the large living room where he was sleeping on the couch, and I noticed that the flames had died down quite a bit. There was just the glow of red hot coals, so I thought I should place another piece of wood on top to keep it going.

When I crept past him there on the couch, I happened to catch a glimpse of him opening his eyes but quickly closing them again. Unfortunately, this was all it took to jumpstart my mind into perceiving he wanted to ignore me. That I was a bother. I was suddenly reliving the old pattern of thought that caused so many heartbreaking moments over the years. I couldn't believe it was happening again. It felt as if I was having some kind of a panic attack where my heart was pounding and even my breathing was affected.

I took a piece of wood and placed it on the coals while trying to remain calm even though my mind was racing out of control. I knew I was having a horrible trigger once again!

Bruce slowly sat up, half asleep.

"What's happening?" he asked.

I was certain he was pretending to be asleep a few seconds ago, which was what caused my mind to crash in the first place! Once it happens, there is no way to avoid reacting (just like when the muscle in the leg suddenly seizes up). I used to call it a brain cramp. The difference was that triggers cause physic pain and are similar in that it happens so fast and so intense that I can't help but react instantly.

I was crushed. It showed I had not been cured—for want of a better word. I felt a rush of anger so strong that it frightened me. I ran into the bedroom and pounded on my pillow till I had no more energy left in my arms. Then I picked up one of the cats that was on the bed and, although gently, actually threw her on the floor as Bruce was coming towards me.

"You just threw Baby out!" he said with a shocked look on his face.

I could see he was deeply disappointed. I think we both knew that the likelihood of our staying together was now next to zero. My mind was reeling with the thought that I was not fixable. At least that was my conclusion.

As he went back to the couch with that all-too-familiar look of *Don't know what to do with her* on his face, I returned to the bedroom and burst into tears as always after a trigger. I beat myself up in my mind for not being able to prevent it. Needless to say, we both felt let down.

We had the best intentions to make our relationship work, and we were planning to get together again when I was ready to leave Le Ricochet. But that episode showed us that I would have to spend more time in Masham. *So I will have to go back,* I thought. I didn't how long I would be there, but I was thankful to have it. And I was glad that Robert happened to be in Montreal and Stephen was at his girlfriend's; at least they were spared the unexpected drama.

I overslept the next morning, which was unusual given that I was always a morning person. Bruce was not in the house. He'd never eaten breakfast since I had known him, so I figured he'd gone to the restaurant where he would have a coffee and read the newspaper, which was his routine. I gathered some clothes and personal items I had come for in the first place while reviewing the previous night's stroll in the backyard.

My heart sank when I realized this was the end for us. There was no choice now; I had to get back to Masham where I could continue with my therapy sessions. *Looks like I still have a lot of work to do in that department,* I thought. *I should wait until Bruce is here first. I want to know exactly what he is thinking.* He's an introvert, so it's not easy to get him to express what's on his mind—as I had learned over the years.

I was sitting in our lovely oak rocking chair next to the large window in the dining area and thinking about how I could make my departure as pleasant as possible, when Bruce came into the circular driveway and stopped right in front of the window. I could see right away from the look on his face that he was struggling with the fact that our relationship was not going the way we had anticipated. I greeted him with a smile, wanting to put him at ease and knowing there would be a certain amount of uncertainty because of the way things had unfolded the night before.

"I'm sorry I woke you up," I said. "And for reacting as I did when I thought you were pretending to be asleep. I was just as surprised as you were, and I realize I definitely will have to spend more time at Le Ricochet for more therapy and healing; so I am ready to leave now, okay?"

He pulled a chair away from the dining room table next to the rocking chair and sat down facing me as if wanting to seriously connect. It was something he never did, so I was curious to hear what he had to say. He hesitated and just stared at me as if searching to find the right words. Then he got and up walked over to the fridge to get a cold drink.

"I've been thinking," he said. "Why not reconsider the idea you had about finding a soulmate—remember? Maybe that would work better for you?"

I knew how difficult it was to actually come out and say it. He must have agonized over having to finally take a stand regarding our relationship. I shouldn't have been surprised since we both saw it was headed in this direction, but even so I couldn't help but feel a stab of emotional pain in that moment.

"I'm not sure what I should do!" I said.

"Well, you spent nine months in Masham and got the professional help you needed," he said with empathy. "Maybe you just need to spend more time there."

"Yes, I will have to go back because the triggers are still there," I said with tears in my eyes. "Guess our expectations were too high. Looks like it will take longer than I thought for me to heal mentally and emotionally, so I'll just have to take it one day at a time and see what happens. At least I know I'm in good hands while I'm there."

So with those final words, disheartening and brief as they were, I put the things I wanted to take back with me into the car and headed back to Masham.

Chapter 22

When I arrived back at Le Ricochet and turned into the driveway, I slowly drove around to the back where my little apartment was at the end. That's when I saw that the portable garage Bruce and Stephen erected for me lying on its side about fifty feet back into the field.

Oh NO! WHAT HAPPENED?

Then it hit me. There must have been a hurricane while I was gone. Sure enough, I found out later that is exactly what happened. I entered my apartment, put my things down and went up to the office, but no one was there. I didn't see anyone else around. *Oh, that's right ... it's Sunday.* As I turned to go back down to put my things away, some writing on the blackboard next to the conference room caught my eye. It read, "Anna Maria's garage is GONE WITH THE WIND!" I couldn't help but laugh even though I was a little upset knowing it would be a job to put it back in place.

The next morning as I was finishing up with my yoga exercises, I heard laughter coming from the hallway. It was unmistakably that of our Louise Beauchemin, so instead of leaving by the back door of my apartment as I normally did to go for my morning walk, I thought I'd go through the hallway and pass by her office. Sure enough, there she was with her usual positive energy.

"Anna Maria! You're back! Wow! I see your garage took a beating with that hurricane!"

"I know, I will call Bruce today to let him know what happened."

"Very good," she said. "It's obvious he really cares about you."

With that, she excused herself and went back to her work. *Hum, she doesn't know that Bruce and I are splitting up for good this time. She'll probably be surprised when she finds out*, I thought. *But I'm not sure about Louise Roy. She seemed to sense even before I went back that we still had some problems to work through should we decide to get back together.*

When I called Bruce to let him know what happened with the garage, he told me not to worry and that he would come back and set it up again.

"I will bring some grey bricks with me this time to secure it properly along the bottom."

I will never forget the many times he came to my rescue when things went wrong; I will be eternally grateful. When he came back again with Stephen the next weekend, I was surprised they were able to get it back up within a short time, but they had to leave soon after. I was not expecting anything more from either of them. Instead, there was this quiet understanding that we would not be getting back together after all. The future was uncertain.

My appointment with Louise Roy was quite interesting. She wanted to know what happened between Bruce and I over the weekend. When I told her in detail what took place, ending with, "Well, it's not like he rejected me," she replied, "In reality that's what it was, a rejection." She helped to clarify our situation by pointing out that the suggestion to find a soulmate was mine in the first place.

"So what Bruce did," she said, "was gently remind you of your own suggestion that you find your so-called soulmate. You are the only one who can decide if that's what you want. But I don't think you should rush into anything just yet. You really need more time to process all that is happening. Overall, though, I find you are doing very well compared to where you were this time last year, don't you think?"

"Yes, things are better now that I have your support, but I am looking forward to the day when I can be free of these triggers and move on with my life."

I noticed a look of concern on her face when I said that, and I wondered, *Does she have doubts about my getting rid of the triggers?*

"Our next appointment will be in my office at the hospital, where I will have someone with me for that particular session. He is a psychiatrist who will determine whether or not you might need some kind of medication, okay?"

I was surprised since I understood the only medication I needed was the hormone pills prescribed by my family doctor when I was in the hospital before going to Le Ricochet.

"Well, I am open to hearing about whatever you have in mind, Louise. After all, it's meant to help me get through this time I have left here at the residence, right?"

So we ended on that note. But I was curious and concerned now. *Does Louise think I will be faced with more problems down the road?*

Ignoring Louise's advice not to rush into anything, I found myself going to Carol, who always kept an eye on how I was doing. He would call me into the conference room whenever he saw I was having a bad day, for instance, and after a fifteen-minute chat I'd always feel much better. So I told him about my intention to find a soulmate to see what he'd say about it.

"It might not be such a bad idea, but I can't help you with that; you're on your own," he said with a chuckle. "He won't come knocking on your door! So you're the one who will have to make the first move, no?"

With that said, I thought, *Why not take a chance, I will never know if I don't give it try.* I knew that Lac Phillippe would no longer be my escape now that the summer season had come to an end and the snow was just around the corner. *In a couple of weeks, I will have been at Le Ricochet for one whole year already.* I realized that what I needed now more than anything was something to focus my attention on before I got caught up with this idea of seeking a soulmate. Around that time, Louise Beauchemin approached me to ask if I would do a picture for Le Ricochet, and I was only too happy to say yes. It was obviously the answer to distract me from rushing into another relationship. The title for my new picture came to me right away, as always happens the moment I chose my subject matter. I decided to call it *Road to Tomorrow*, and I threw myself into creating this expression, which would take at least five weeks to complete in addition to the framing.

As always when I worked on my art, I had to limit my time to no more than two hours or else I'd get pain in my head. Even so, those two hours a day were enough to keep my mind from wandering off into the wrong direction during the winter months. Taking the time each day to get out for morning walks, as well as getting my meditation and yoga exercises in along with my artwork, enabled me to put my concerns regarding the future on hold. I took it one day at a time as I had planned.

I was worried about how I would manage being inside again with the other residents during the cold weather. When I first arrived, I did not do so well when we were gathered there at the dining table. When Louise moved me into my own apartment, it was a blessing in disguise, I suppose. Even so, there was always a certain amount of interaction since we were all living under the same roof. The other residents were not aware that I suffered from triggers, so I was always on guard and hoping to avoid any problem. But I found this to be stressful at times. Consequently, I tried to be alone as much as possible to avoid any incidents.

One day while totally absorbed in my artwork, there was a knock on my door. It was Louise Beauchemin wanting to see how I was doing with the picture for Le Ricochet.

"If you don't mind, Anna Maria, I would like to show your art to my guests who are here from east Asia."

"Sure, no problem," I said.

When she stepped inside my apartment, she was followed by four gentlemen, each one bowing slightly in a gesture of greeting as they came in. I showed them the few framed pieces I had hung on the wall as well as the one I was currently working on.

"Umm … aahh," they murmured, smiling and nodding politely as if genuinely interested in my work; a rather charming reflection of their culture.

"I'm giving them a tour of our complex to see first-hand how we run our residence here in Quebec," Louise said. "So I'll take them around our newly renovated building now!"

They appeared enthusiastic and curious, wanting to see everything there at Le Ricochet. It was a real pleasure just to meet with them.

I went to the hospital for my appointment with Louise Roy as she had instructed. While waiting to be called, I happened to be sitting under the sign "Mental Heath," and I remember feeling self-conscious, probably because of the stigma associated with mental illness. But I relaxed when the door to her office opened and she greeted me warmly, as always. A man whom I presumed to be the psychiatrist that she mentioned was sitting next to her desk.

"Hello, I'm Dr. Andre Aubin," he said, standing up to shake my hand and then pointing to the empty chair for me to sit down.

Louise sat behind her desk with her files open as if they had been discussing my case already. I expected he would start talking to me when I sat down, but Louise carried on with our session as she normally did. On that particular day, she happened to be talking about how I was interacting with some of the residents. She pointed out my having had some conflict and made a suggestion as to how I should go about avoiding such problems in the future.

"You might want to change your approach," she said. "People don't like to be told what to do."

"Yes, I understand what you're saying Louise," I replied.

"Evidently, everything is either black or white for you—there are no grey areas. Maybe we could pick up on this during our next appointment," she said, indicating our session was finished.

"Are you aware, Anna Maria, that you jump from one subject to another in the middle of a conversation?" Dr. Aubin asked with a curious look.

"Really? No, actually, I didn't realize I did that."

Then after I said a few more things, he added, "Perfectionism isn't easy, is it?"

I gathered from that remark that I must be a perfectionist, which didn't surprise me because I am forever trying to do things better—raising the bar, so to speak. At the end of our session when he was about to get up to leave, he leaned over and looked me straight in the eye.

"You know, you could write a book," he said. When I laughed, he said, "I'm serious; you could write a book."

Louise must have told him about my life. His words and the way he looked at me with such conviction when he said it, must have registered in the back of my mind. Because this idea of writing a book actually did pop up in my mind over the years until I finally decided to give it a try, like, decades later. At the end of our session that day, Dr. Aubin suggested I take some pills to help me get through that rough period when I couldn't sleep at night.

At my first yearly check-up with Dr. Folkerson, he made an interesting analogy which helped me to accept my condition and not be so hard on myself.

"You seem to think it's your fault that you have these triggers," he said as he reached for my file. "You shouldn't blame yourself."

I was in awe of his deep understanding and empathy, something I definitely wasn't used to.

"Your 'environment and emotional state' have a lot to do with your mental condition. For example, when a person with asthma suffers an attack, these two factors play a huge part."

Then he helped me more than he realized when he said, "If you think you can't handle your situation at the residence at any given time, know you can always come into the hospital for a day or two. I will advise Louise Beauchemin on this as well."

That profound statement kept running through my mind over and over as I drove back to the residence. Knowing that I would not be kicked out if a trigger occurred made me feel less apprehensive about the coming weeks—or possibly months—that I would be living there. Even so, I knew I had to be extra careful when connecting with the residents and caregivers alike.

Chapter 23

Time passed by quickly as I entered into my second year at Le Ricochet. The Christmas party had come and gone already, and I finished my picture as I had planned. There was always something going on to help keep everyone occupied, which I really liked.

I had an unexpected visit from Louise with pen and cheque book in hand, asking how much I wanted for my picture.

"No, I won't charge for it, Louise. I want to give it as a donation."

When she insisted, I gave in; she certainly had a way with persuasion. She then told me about a fashion show she had planned to raise funds for Le Ricochet and asked if I'd be interested in participating.

"I'll think about it," I said, as it sounded rather interesting.

I ended up sitting in the audience instead, happily soaking up the exciting vibes as the participants clearly enjoyed strutting their stuff. One of the participants was a slim, attractive young woman who came out smiling and looking so confident in her sporty outfit with matching shirt, shorts and baseball cap. Normally she was quite reserved, so I was delighted to see how this experience helped her, along with the others, to express themselves in such a positive way.

I was so busy I even forgot about my soulmate search until the idea surfaced again in that spring of 1999. I happened to be working on another picture I wanted to donate of a woman sitting and gazing out at a sailboat on the lake. I used the sailboat because it was a logo for Le Ricochet. I continued to stay centred and focused on my art and was determined to keep it that way. At the same time, though, I couldn't seem to let go of this fantasy to find someone I could share my life with when I eventually left Le Ricochet.

Every once in a while, I'd get a call from either Bruce or Robert wanting to know how things were going, which I appreciated since I had not been in touch with anyone for quite some time. When Bruce asked if I had made any progress in finding a soulmate, I said, "No, I am keeping myself busy so as not to rush into anything on the advice of my psychotherapist, Louise Roy."

But then after my conversation with him, I thought maybe it was time to pick up on that again now that I felt I was almost ready to leave and be on my own. I really did believe there might be someone out there who was searching for me as well. My mental health had improved, at least in my opinion, because there were no problems relating to triggers for quite some time. I took this as a sign to move forward no matter what the others thought.

As I had expected, there were no positive reactions from the residents. One man even said, "You're past your prime, do you really think you're going to find someone at your age?" I thought it was a rude thing to say, but it made me even more determined, and I jotted down the words: "Let's see what Ba Ba will do!" on a piece of paper and stuck it on my door. He was aware I used this term as an affectionate name for the Supreme, so I put it where he couldn't miss it. However, the staff, administration and caregivers were more open to my endeavour, and they showed some interest and even a little support. Julie happened to be on duty that day and overheard his disparaging remark. She immediately came to my defence with compliments regarding my positive spirit and how well I took care of myself.

I placed a very small ad in the companions column of the *Wakefield News* saying I was interested in a long-term relationship. I had only three replies in the mail. The first one I chose to answer was rather interesting, however, it was not what I had expected. When we met at a restaurant in Wakefield over brunch, I knew within minutes that this connection was not meant to be. I didn't keep him for long before I politely told him I had to leave so as not to mislead him in any way, and we parted ways.

Then I thought, *Why don't I reach out farther and try the* Ottawa Citizen *newspaper?* Cheryl and Clair, both caregivers whom I had a close relationship with, agreed with me on that, so I went ahead and placed the ad. I had seven or eight replies, two of which stood out as possible connections; they both lived in Ottawa West. The first one I called came to meet with me in Wakefield in front of the General Store as I had suggested. While waiting in my car, I couldn't help but recall that it was where I found Lora's ad on the bulletin board the first time I came to Wakefield and where I ate the tomato and bun while sitting at the water's edge, stressed out and in terrible pain. I couldn't help but see how much things had improved. I was now free of the pain and was becoming more confident than I had ever been.

As I sat there, the high-pitched sound of a train whistle suddenly caught my attention as the Ottawa/Wakefield tourist train slowly came into view and stopped right there next to the General Store. I always loved the sight, sound and feel of that magnificent steam train; it turned out to be a wonderful surprise that day.

Moments later, a car pulled up close to mine and the driver got out, paused and looked around. I figured it was my date, so I stepped out. We exchanged greetings and since it was such a beautiful sunny day, I suggested we stroll along with everyone else as they disembarked from the train and made their way into the lovely shops along the river. From there, we decided to drop into a cozy little restaurant to have a bite. After a short brunch, I thought, *Why not invite him to come and see my art since he is interested.* Carol was on duty that day and told me it would be okay.

I knew the caregivers were curious, but they were also looking out for me, which I appreciated very much. Unfortunately, the polite manners he had displayed prior to coming into my apartment disappeared while I was explaining what each expression hanging on the wall meant for me.

He caught me off guard when he put his arm around my waist and pulled me close, trying to kiss me. I politely let him know I was not comfortable with his sudden advances, but he persisted anyway. That's when I became annoyed.

"I'm sorry, but I am no longer interested in pursuing this any further," I said, "so maybe you should leave now."

He appeared to be insulted, so I took a moment to persuade him to simply leave without further incident. I knew I had made the right decision but was a little embarrassed when I told Carol about it shortly afterwards.

"Oh well, there's other fish in the sea, as they say. Don't you have other replies?" he asked.

"Yes, as a matter of fact there is another one in Ottawa that I'm interested in as well, so hopefully that one will have a more positive outcome."

That evening I read his reply over a few more times. It said he was interested in having a long-term monogamous relationship, so I went up to use the phone in the conference room where it was more private. I connected with a gentleman whose name was David. When I heard his voice, I immediately felt at ease as he described what he was looking for in a relationship.

"By the way, I didn't mention in my reply that I have a fifteen year old son who alternates between living with me and his mother, whose house is only one street over from where I live," he added in an apologetic tone. "I preferred to tell you about this in person in case it might deter you from responding."

"I have no problem with that at all," I said. "Actually, it's good that you're being up front with me, and I can assure you I will definitely do the same."

After exchanging basic information, I asked what he thought about meeting up for brunch that coming Sunday, which just happened to be Mother's Day. He said he'd be delighted, so we talked a little more and decided on a place and time to meet up.

My plan was to meet in front of the General Store as I did with the other person, and then stroll along the path at the water's edge to chat some more before going to the restaurant. This time, I chose Earl's House, which was on the corner of the T-intersection where you come down the hill into Wakefield. I was quite satisfied with my conversation with David, and we'd shared much more information over the phone before our meeting than I had with the previous connections.

Falling asleep took a while that night. Anticipation turned into excitement the more I thought about what a special weekend this might turn out to be for both of us. I really did like his voice, among other things. He mentioned he enjoyed cooking and that he thought about being a chef.

"But that was way back when," he said.

We shared a lot over the phone, and now we would see what happens as the weekend unfolded. I hoped he would find something to make him want to see me again, but I wanted to keep my expectations low.

There was something I picked up on during our phone conversation which made me curious. Not only was Mother's Day on May 9, but that year happened to be 1999. Plus the address of Le Ricochet 9 Chemin Burriere. I noted a major change had occurred in both of our lives at the tender age of nine as well. It was when his parents brought him, his brother and his sister over from England, and that's the age I was when Papa suddenly passed away. It was fascinating that this number kept popping up, and it was compelling enough to make me want to learn more.

By the time Sunday morning rolled around, I had convinced myself that he was that special someone, and I was a little nervous. But I couldn't wait to meet up with him face to face.

When I arrived early, there were three vehicles parked next to the General Store. One of them was a blue van, and he mentioned he'd be driving one as well. I didn't see anyone inside when I pulled up next to it. *Hum … maybe it's not David's.* That's when the figure of a man walking on the railroad tracks next to the store caught my eye. I got out of my car and, with a closer look, saw he fit the description. White hair with short beard, glasses, blue shirt—that must be him! *So we're both early this morning; a good sign*, I thought.

He was looking down, stepping carefully as he walked along the railroad tracks, so he didn't see me coming. I wanted to call his name but chose to walk over instead. As I approached him from behind, I noticed he had rather broad shoulders.

"David?" I asked in an inquisitive tone.

I obviously startled him, so I apologized. He was holding a thermos and looked slightly confused, as if not sure how to react.

"Would it be okay with you if we just sit here by the water and have a coffee before going to the restaurant?" he asked.

This was totally unexpected. I hesitated since there was no one else around and there were low-lying bushes. *Is this safe?* I must say, though, he appeared to be a real gentleman and seemed quite sincere with his intentions. But then I thought, *No I shouldn't take the risk*.

"Maybe it would be better if we just go to the restaurant sooner rather than later?"

"It's up to you," he replied.

"Okay, they should be open by now. Being Mother's Day, it will be busy so I reserved a table for us," I said.

As we walked to our vehicles, he took my hand in his as if wanting to simply reassure me because I think he noticed I had become a little tense at his suggestion of coffee first. From there the energy changed and I felt more relaxed when we both got into our vehicles and headed for the restaurant just down the street.

It was one of those large older houses with a veranda wrapped around the building that had a beautiful view of the lake. Each table had a candle with a beautiful long stemmed red rose placed next to it, adding that special touch. David was courteous and open with me. When they rolled the little cart of food over to our table, David stood up, and taking one of the platters, asked, "So what would you like?"

"Well, I am a vegetarian, so I will avoid the meat, of course."

"Okay, now I know what not to cook for you," he said with a smile.

We were getting to know quite a bit about each other, and I was comfortable just being there with him. We went on to enjoy a wonderful brunch together, and I showed him a few pictures of my art as well. I asked if he'd like to come and see where I lived since it was only ten minutes away from Wakefield. I did not mention my mental condition or that I was living at Le Ricochet just yet. I was anxious about it because I wanted to see his reaction in person as opposed to telling him over the phone. Now that we were together, I was still hesitant to talk about it because I feared it would turn him away, I guess, so I kept putting it off. *I'll tell him when he's about to leave*, I thought. That way he could think it over when he got home and then make up his mind as to whether or not he wanted to see me again.

We both seemed satisfied with the way things were going, and when we left the restaurant, he followed behind as we drove towards Masham. He did look a little puzzled as we got out of our vehicles at Le Ricochet, but he didn't ask any questions. I invited him in to see my art, which he seemed to like, then we just talked together.

We were there maybe an hour or so when I finally sensed it was the right time to bring up the mental health issue. I was terribly apprehensive, but it was past my time to rest and knew if I didn't do that I'd end up with pain in my head. By then my nervousness was beginning to show.

"Are you okay?" he asked.

"Well, I did say I would be as up front with you as you have been with me, so I'm trying to find a way to tell you something you should know before you leave."

"Yes, I believe we are being open and honest with each other, which I think we should be," he said with a slight grin.

The undercurrent of fear I had of being rejected took over and made it almost impossible to come out and say what I wanted to express.

"Well … as you can see for yourself, I am living in this group home," I said. "I have been here for over a year, but I expect to be out on my own within a few months. I'm sure you're wondering why I'm here, so I will briefly explain my current situation, okay?"

"Yes, I am want to hear what you have to say, Anna Maria."

He said it with such a sincere expression that my anxiety instantly decreased. It also gave me the impression that he just might be able to absorb and process what I was about to reveal without judgment. This had been my major concern. How was he going to handle this information regarding my mental condition? I managed to find enough courage to divulge my "secret."

"So, why don't we sit at the table and have a tea before you go?" I suggested.

"Why not, I'm in no hurry," he replied in a rather charming way that let me know he wasn't about to bail out—not just yet anyway.

He appeared curious to know what was on my mind. I just wanted to get it over with, so I dove in.

"I came here for help after experiencing a mental breakdown a year and a half ago. It happened a few months after I broke up with my husband whom I had been with for twenty-seven years. I left my marriage thinking I would be able make it on my own, but unfortunately that didn't happen. Thankfully, this place has made it possible for me to receive the best of care, regular therapy sessions and some space to let the healing process take place with each passing day."

I was extremely nervous, and I abruptly brought my account to a close with a rather flippant remark: "So that's it in a nutshell! You must be on overload by now anyway."

I wanted to see his reaction, but I felt much too vulnerable, so I quickly got up and gently placed my chair at the table.

"I know this is a lot for you to take in, David, so I'm sure you will need some time to process it all. Now if you don't mind, we'll just call it a day; what do you say?"

He stood up with a surprised look that told me I was probably being too abrupt, maybe even a little rude, so I said, "I really would like to spend more time with you, David, but I have to take some time to rest now." Apparently he understood that I didn't want to just get rid of him because that's when he picked up the newspaper, walked over to the rocking chair and sat down. This was a clear indication to me that I was not about to be rejected because of my mental condition, which was huge. Plus, he obviously didn't need time to think this over; he had every intention of sticking around despite the possibility there could be challenges ahead.

"So this has turned out to be an exceptional Mother's Day, thanks to you, David," I said. "I really did enjoy our time together at Earl's House."

"Actually I didn't expect to come back with you," he said, "but I'm glad I did, and I appreciate the way you are being so candid with me."

"Well, I see you're in no hurry to leave. Maybe you'd like to read the newspaper while I have a cat nap?"

"Sure, I'm quite comfortable here," he replied.

"I appreciate the way you're honouring my request in the ad that I was looking for a relationship based on trust and respect," I said.

It was obvious that we shared the same values, and he read the newspaper while I was resting. This was one of the characteristics he had displayed which I liked very much. It was sufficient enough to erase any doubts I had when we first met in front of the General Store that day.

David turned out to be a complete gentleman. We chatted for another hour or so after my half-hour rest, and then as he was about to leave, he asked if he could see me again. I was more than happy to say yes. A few seconds later there was a gentle knock on the door and David poked his head inside.

"I just want to say I find your art to be very interesting," he said.

Then he waved goodbye as he turned and walked towards his van.

I immediately went to talk to Cheryl.

"So? How did it go this time?" she asked with wide-eyed anticipation.

"Well, that's what I want to tell you about," I said, bubbling with excitement. "He was very much the gentleman, showing nothing but total respect. Maybe you could let me know if I'm getting a little ahead of myself when I say this, but I do believe I have found my soulmate—like today! Mother's Day! Can you believe it? Since it's still sunny outside, I think I'll go for a walk. When I get back, if you're interested, I'll share the details with you, okay?"

"Absolutely—can't wait to hear all about it!"

So off I went feeling positive and uplifted after having the most incredible Mother's Day ever. After being on a spiritual path for so many years, I couldn't help but see this through a spiritual lens. The Supreme Being, our creator, is the one who ultimately makes all our connections.

As I left the residence, I chose to go in the opposite direction of where I would normally go for my morning walks because there was this farm about a mile down the road where I often saw a couple of horses in the field. Today I thought why not go that way for a change, and I wondered if the horses would still be there. Sure enough, as I came within sight of the farm, there they were, grazing right next to the cedar fence. One was a gorgeous dark rust colour with a blond mane and tail, and the other was beautifully speckled grey. They were those strong, beautiful workhorses with the big hooves, and I wanted to get close enough to pet them. As I walked over to the fence, their ears perked up and they walked towards me. I grabbed a handful of grass and stretched my arm out over the fence, offering it to them as they came closer. I think they were expecting something more appealing than a handful of grass because they quickly lost interest once they they discovered it was all I had in my hand. At least I was able to pat and stroke them for those few minutes, which made me happy. It reminded me of the team we had back home when I was a child.

I was simply enjoying the moment, and I couldn't resist picking a bunch of daisies that were growing alongside the fence to take back with me. I put them in a little vase and placed it on the dining room table before sitting down with Cheryl to share my day's experience.

I couldn't imagine things getting any better than they were. I ended my day feeling nothing but pure gratitude that my situation had improved tenfold since I'd left Saint-Jean-de-Matha a year and a half before. *Hum … what will psychotherapist Louise have to say about all this?* I wondered. I remembered I had an appointment with her in a few days' time.

As I tucked myself into bed that night, the phone rang. To my surprise it was David. I didn't expect to hear from him so soon, so I was elated to hear his voice. He was more or less updating me on what happened with the rest of his day, and then he asked about mine. He said he took his mother, who was in her nineties, and his fifteen-year-old son out for dinner that evening. He also wanted me to know he would be coming up to see me again on the weekend.

"What do you think about having a little picnic at Lac Philippe in the Gatineau Park while you're here, since it's only a two-minute drive from the residence?"

"That sounds like a great idea, I would love that," he said.

"Okay, so I will make my own vegetarian burgers and a salad, and we should have a really nice time at the lake."

"I will get in touch with you by the middle of the week," he said.

That phone call, which lasted only a few minutes, left no doubt in my mind. We definitely had a good connection. We had already shared a lot in such a short time, and I felt confident that everything would workout. I was tempted to give Robert a call just then to let him know, but I changed my mind because he would be concerned, as usual; I didn't want him to worry for nothing. Besides, you never know. Even though things appear to be perfect, all could change in an instant as I have learned over the years. I couldn't help but recall the times when I was totally lost out there in the world, taking so many chances with no backup whatsoever. But now with some support behind me, I was pretty sure I'd be able to handle anything that came my way. I felt stronger than ever.

That Mother's Day had turned out to be so very special that it sparked my imagination and inspired another creation. I gave it the title *To Our Future Together*. But then I thought maybe I should wait. It was better not to get ahead of myself, so I put it on hold.

Louise Beauchemin was back in her office Monday morning, and she asked about my weekend with David. She said Cheryl had mentioned it to her, and I could see she was happy for me even though she didn't say so herself.

When I saw Louise Roy the next day, she, of course, wanted to know what was happening with the ad I'd placed. This was the person I really wanted to share my experience with because I knew she would be straightforward and point out whatever I should think twice about. I started out careful with my words so as not to give her any reason to find a problem, but once I started talking, I just let it all out. I knew she'd read between the lines anyway.

"Well, when I finally told David about my condition, it wasn't easy because I remembered Dr. Folkerson advising me to wait a while before telling anyone about my mental health problem. As it turned out, I didn't do that.

I wanted to know his reaction even though it was our first date, so I went ahead and told him just before he left that Sunday. I know it's too soon to know for sure, but I can't help thinking that he's 'the one.'"

"Well, you are right about it being too soon to know," Louise said. "I am very interested in hearing more when you come back in two weeks time, and we'll take it from there, okay?"

I was hoping for some feedback, but she obviously wasn't ready to make any comment or suggestion. I figured she wanted to wait until I had more to share, so I would have to wait.

David brought the best wine and cheese, which made our picnic that much more special. He shared that he lived on the top floor of a duplex with his son who alternates between living with him and his ex-wife. His elderly mother had lived on the main floor by herself ever since her husband passed away. She'd had a stroke that left her legally blind and walking with a cane, so David helped to take care of her by coming home from work when he could to make lunch for her.

He seemed like such an exceptional person. He was totally up front beginning with his first marriage to a school teacher. He said they had no problems until she got pregnant and had their firstborn. Unfortunately, she suffered from post-partum depression right after their baby was born. She wouldn't talk to anyone, not even with her parents whom she got along with just fine before the depression hit. Then without any warning, she surprised everyone by taking the baby and moving to another province. David hadn't seen or heard from either of them since.

Later on, he married again, but she did not want to have any children in the year and a half that they were together. Finally, his most recent marriage was with the mother of his now fifteen-year-old son, Alexis. She already had a six-year-old daughter named Sylvie when they got married, he said.

After hearing his marriage history, I decided to let him know about my own relationships. We cleared the air, so to speak, by addressing this topic that would have to be discussed sooner or later. I felt good about taking care of that sooner, and now we could move on with getting to know each other better.

I invited David into the residence to give him a tour of the complex after the picnic. Just then, Clair, the mayor's wife, arrived for her evening shift. She was her usual joyful self, making us both feel comfortable, which I appreciated very much.

After David left, Clair happened to be sitting in the living room watching TV since some of the residents were away for the weekend and it was pretty quiet. She wasn't busy and seemed open to having a conversation.

"Would you like to come and sit down, Anna Maria?" she asked.

"Okay, but not for long because it's time to have my rest," I said.

"I'm glad I had a chance to meet David today," she said. "He seems like a very nice man."

"Yes, I know. We talked about our past relationships today on our picnic at Lac Philippe, so we're getting to know quite a bit about each other in a short time. Both of us are trying to be as transparent as possible."

She asked if he had been married before, and when I said he has three ex-wives, she jumped up with a shocked look on her face and said, "Oh NO, Anna Maria! Really?" It was as if she was afraid I was making a big mistake.

I laughed and said, "Do you know how many times I was married, Clair?"

"I know you were married to Bruce for over twenty-years," she said.

"But that wasn't my only marriage; actually, I've had as many as David."

She sat down again, still looking concerned and slightly embarrassed for reacting so strongly.

"I know you have my best interests at heart, but I have a history when it comes to relationships that you're not aware of," I said.

"So you talked about that with him today and think there's no cause for concern?" she asked.

"Well, yes, but for the most part we are on the same page when it comes to being cautious this time around. With all that we've experienced over the years, we do not intend to repeat mistakes. Even though we're both in our fifties, I am optimistic and believe it's not too late to find happiness in a lasting relationship."

As I got up to leave, she said, "I commend you for having the courage, and I hope it all works out for you."

"Thank you, Clair. I really am feeling positive about everything and don't think there is anything to worry about. So I'll have my rest now and will see you after supper, okay?"

So as not to appear too anxious, I waited for David to call me during the week as he said he would. But when he contacted me on Wednesday night and asked me to meet his family that coming weekend, I surprised myself by suddenly putting the brakes on. I realized that I had built up my confidence by telling myself I was ready for anything, but the reality was … I wasn't! So I quickly searched for some excuse to put it off for now.

"Umm … what do you think if we had lunch at Earl's House in Wakefield this weekend instead and maybe I could go to Ottawa to meet your family another time?" I asked.

"Well, if that's what you prefer, then I'll come up to Wakefield on Sunday," he said.

I hoped he wouldn't misunderstand my reluctance to go, so when I saw him on the weekend, I explained my hesitations; he understood, as I had hoped he would.

I was finally able to put my insecurities aside and meet with his family the next weekend. His mother, Florence, although in her nineties, was alert and welcoming. With her lovely English accent, she said, "Come and join us for dinner, dear," as she walked with her cane to take her place at the table in the dining room. David's fifteen-year-old son Alexis was there with Mitzi, David's sister. The table had a lovely setting with a fresh bouquet of flowers for a centrepiece, and as we sat down Florence placed a small, framed picture next to the flowers. David said it was a photo of his father who had passed away a few years ago. *Oh, how sweet to have his picture there on the table,* I thought.

They were not only very sociable, but everyone shared interesting conversations. It was quite pleasant, but at the same time I noticed Alexis was not comfortable with my presence. Although this triggered a feeling of rejection in my mind, I was able to get through dinner without showing how much I was struggling. I couldn't wait to get back to my to apartment on Monday where I would feel emotionally safe. It took a lot of effort to get past those feelings, and I didn't say anything to David. I hoped I'd quickly get over this little stumbling block that was in the way.

It was sad how terribly insecure I was at that time. If a five-year-old had looked at me sideways, it would have affected me. Even though it wasn't apparent to others, I had a difficult time being close to anyone whom I felt did not want to connect with me.

A few weeks later when I went back to Ottawa with David, we stopped in to see Flo before going upstairs to his place. Alexis happened to be staying at his mother's house, so I felt more comfortable. Florence was very welcoming again, and she actually seemed eager to have a conversation. Before we left, she offered us tickets to a play at the Ottawa Little Theatre. She was a lifetime member there and had tickets for every show. She even had a seat with her name tag on it.

I found out she used to act on stage with William Shatner before he went to Hollywood and became famous as Captain Kirk in *Star Trek*. They kept in touch. Flo stayed in Ottawa doing what she loved most, performing on stage as a leading lady, up until she suffered a stroke and had to leave the profession altogether. I was delighted to have met her, and I let David know it, but I was a little skeptical about Alexis. I was concerned the situation might be a challenge for me down the road.

"So I'm curious about your late father," I said one day. "I got the impression your mother is quite fond of him. What kind of a relationship did you have with him? Were you close?"

"Yes, he taught me a lot, and we really do miss having him here with us. He was an architect and worked for the federal government when we came over from England. He designed the monument with the eternal flame on Parliament Hill, along with the large globe structure close by at Rideau Falls. Later on, he worked in his own architectural business until he passed away from a massive heart attack in his mid-eighties. One of the reasons my parents loved being involved with the Ottawa Little Theatre was that he designed it as well."

"Did you have any interest in the theatre yourself, David?"

"No, not in the way my mother did, but as a teenager I liked helping my dad when he worked on the stagecraft, and I enjoyed doing the sound and lighting here and at another theatre called the Brey Manor just outside Montreal. That's where my mother spent her summers when she was acting on stage outside of Ottawa. Actually, I intended to go to Pasadena, California, to study theatre arts but it turned out to be too expensive. That's when a friend of my parents suggested I apply for a job at Crawley Films, Canada's largest independent film producer. I worked there for a number of years until it finally closed. Right after that, I decided to go with a few film technicians to the United States where we were hired to work for the North Carolina State Film Board."

"So what brought you back to Ottawa?"

"I didn't stay in the US because of the situation with the Vietnam War at that time, so I changed my mind and came back home."

"You have experience in a number of work situations, so what did you do when you returned to Ottawa?"

"I worked for a number of years in the imported car business before deciding to open up a dealership of my own. Maybe I'll just fast forward here to when I had my RV service here in Westboro. That's when I was asked if I'd sell my property so that a three-tower condominium complex could be erected on the sight. When the deal went through, the owner wanted me to work for him, which I agreed to do, and I have been there ever since. It was a good move because I enjoy interacting with the people living in the complex as well as with the business owners there."

"And to be living close to where you work is an advantage, I would think, along with it being in such a lovely neighbourhood."

"I've spent most of my life in this area, and I do like living here."

"It's too bad I didn't get to meet your father," I said. "I would like to get to know the rest of your family, but because of my mental condition, I will have to take it slow, especially with Alexis. I sense he may be having a problem accepting me as your new partner, and I can understand that. Maybe after he gets to know me, he'll be more receptive? By the way, how is the arrangement working out with him spending time at both places?"

"It looks as if he has adjusted reasonably well; I haven't had any complaints about it so far. I really don't think we have anything to worry about; I'm pretty sure he'll adapt to the situation in time, and everything will work for all of us."

Chapter 24

That spring and summer, I was preoccupied with making sure this new relationship with David didn't suddenly go off the rails. I was constantly worried that a misunderstanding between us could trigger some emotions that might surprise him (and me). Actually, our relationship seemed too good to be true when I got through that summer without any major problems, not only with David, but with the other residents as well. It was probably because I was so careful to avoid contact with them; I was still quite sensitive to any signs of rejection, but it looked as if my strategy worked well.

When I started to go to David's house about every second weekend, I thought I'd reconnect with the margii family, since they happened to live close by. I began to spend time there for kiirtan (the dance we always do just before meditation). Robert and Bruce had kept in touch, leaving me with a good sense of connection during that time. I was also fortunate enough to get away whenever things got tense for me at the residence by simply going over to the lake, as I did the previous summer.

I noted how all these factors added up and made it possible for my healing to continue. My therapy sessions with Louise Roy were essential in helping me to move forward. She gradually understood why I was so adamant about David being my soulmate, and she agreed to have him come along to one of my appointments.

He sat quietly during our session, and as we were about to leave, she said, "Well, Anna Maria, we already know you suffer from triggers, now we have to find out what causes them."

The positive way in which she interacted with both of us left me feeling reassured, and David was very supportive, providing encouragement whenever needed. It wasn't long before I realized just how much I had come to rely on his emotional support.

On David's next visit to Le Ricochet, he brought a thick white binder. He placed it on the table and the word NAMI stood out. The cover read: "Open your mind … mental illnesses are brain disorders." I was curious, of course.

"What's this?" I asked.

"I want to show you something," he said. "I started to take this family-to-family educational program with NAMI, the National Alliance for the Mentally Ill. I will attend on a weekly basis for a couple of months."

I was dumbfounded. I really did not know what to say. He was obviously taking this course to have a deeper understanding of mental illness. It was crystal clear to me now just how much he truly cared. This had a huge impact on me both mentally and emotionally. There was no doubt left in my mind—David was truly the soulmate I had been searching for. I began to call him my guardian angel as well as my earth angel, which he seemed to genuinely like.

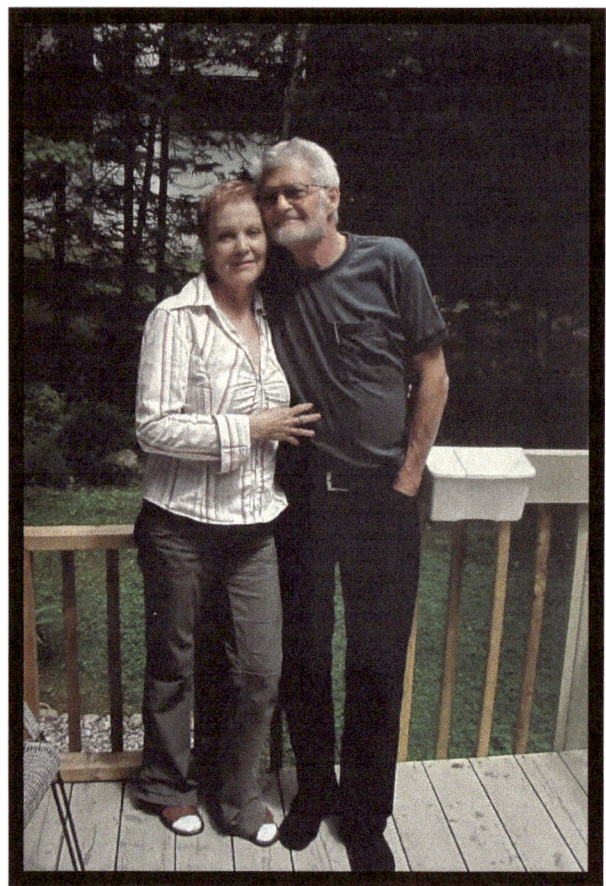

SOUL-MATES DAVID AND ANNA MARIA

A few months later, David and I attended an event that Louise Beauchemin had organized. As she sat down at the table across from us, she jokingly remarked, "Looks like David is your little miracle, Anna Maria!" We laughed, but deep down I knew this to be true because I saw it through the lens of a spiritual aspirant.

Louise had arranged for me to share my latest piece of artwork at the event. It would be showcased that evening and would be the only piece of art on display. I must say it did get a lot of attention. I had it mounted in a shiny gold frame and placed it on an easel. A little plaque was attached, and I covered it with a cloth so it could be unveiled during dinner.

When it was time to introduce my work, I froze for a second when I was handed the microphone. I was a little embarrassed because my French wasn't up to par. I began with "Bonjour everyone," then immediately switched to English to explain the meaning of this particular expression titled *Road to Tomorrow*. It depicted two figures (from behind) from the waist up who were moving along this long, winding road. There was a large question mark in the foreground to show how uncertain the future looks when one is struggling with a mental disorder. I made my speech as short as possible, saying we don't know where this road to tomorrow leads, but we can still dream and believe that, despite the challenges, life is still worth living.

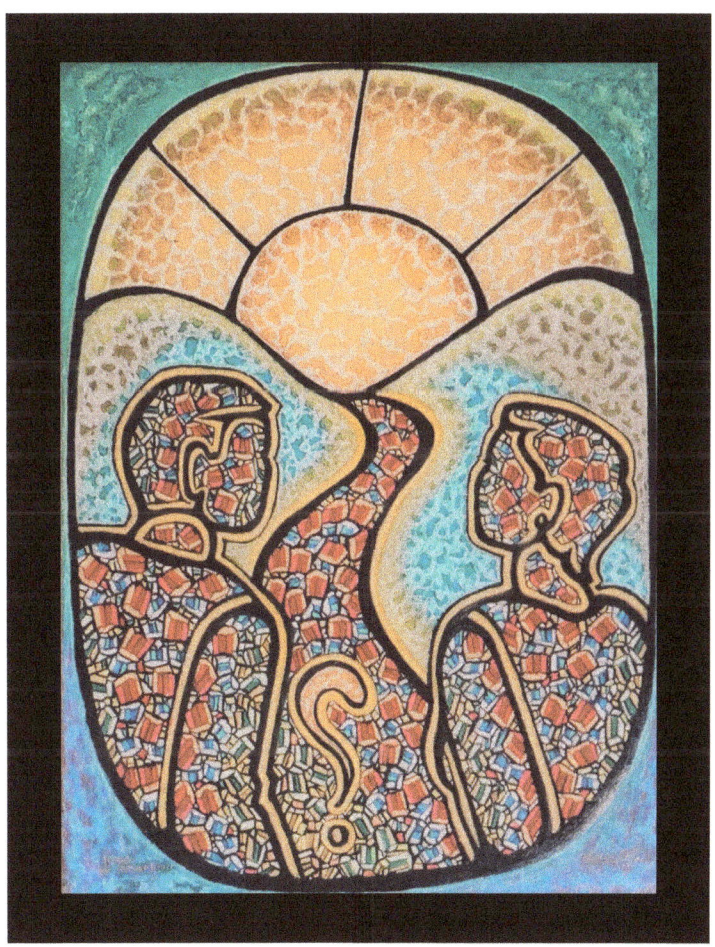

ROAD TO TOMORROW

I handed the mic back to the MC and heard her thanking me as I scurried back to our table. On my way, I was startled when someone reached out and grabbed my hand as I passed by. I paused for a moment and her eyes welled up as she expressed how she was touched by what I had said.

"You're giving hope to those struggling with mental conditions," she said.

I guess I was so wrapped up in trying to just get through that evening without making a complete fool of myself that I didn't even think about how my words might have resonated with some of the people there. Just to know I actually had something to offer that evening ultimately helped me to understand something about myself. I was slowly discovering that I may not be as worthless a person as I thought. It was a step forward in my evolution in consciousness.

Chapter 25

By 2000, I was into my third year at Le Ricochet, so I was sort of expecting it when Louise Beauchemin called me into her office to discuss my situation. She was rather upbeat about it.

"Anna Maria! I was just on the phone with a neighbour who has a furnished basement apartment to rent. Would you like to go and have a look at it today?"

"For sure!" I replied. "I've been looking around trying to find something I can afford. Actually, Julie has been helping me with this," I said.

"Well, I'm sure you won't be disappointed with this place. It has two large bedrooms, is completely furnished and is very clean. They're only charging $400 a month."

"Really? Sounds great! The last place I checked out charged $500 a month."

"The couple renting this place are very particular when it comes to their tenants," she said. "Both are retired. She was a school teacher here, and her husband was the principal. We think it would be perfect for you; you won't feel alone because the door to upstairs is always open. I was told they come down once in a while just to water the plants and put food into their freezer. And it's very quiet, so as you're an artist, we thought it would be the best possible place for you."

"This sounds too good to be true, Louise. I can't wait to see it!"

"Great! I'll call them back to tell them you're on your way over, okay? It's only a few minutes away. Here's the address; their names are Suzanne and Raymond, a lovely couple."

As we entered the house from downstairs, I followed behind Raymond. I didn't realize it was the apartment at first because it appeared to be part of their living quarters when we stepped inside. But when he stopped and asked, "So, what do you think?" I looked around at what appeared to be a large living room with beautiful hanging plants and lovely furniture.

"Is this it?" I asked.

"Yes," he replied.

I was amazed. It was not any average apartment and they were charging much less than the other places I'd seen. There were two couches with end tables, lovely hanging plants and a modern potbelly gas stove had a cozy fire burning behind its glass window. A sliding glass door to the patio was at the end of the kitchen cupboards, and on the right side of the stairs leading up to the main floor was the bathroom and two large bedrooms.

Granted, it wasn't totally private, but it was much more than I could have dreamed of given my situation at the time. I had such problems in the previous few weeks trying to find a place that I was starting to get a little discouraged. This was a godsend.

"This is absolutely beautiful!" I said. "So when can I move in?"

"It is ready whenever you are," he replied. "It has been empty since a relative stayed here while visiting from out west last year."

I put two and two together and figured Louise was instrumental in finding this place for me. Overcome with gratitude, I went straight to her office.

"Thank you so much, Louise!" I said as I was leaving" And thank you, Ba Ba!"

"Don't thank Ba Ba! Thank Raymond and Suzanne for renting the place!" she quipped.

The next day when I was gathering my belongings together, someone tapped on my half-open door.

"Anna Maria?" Carol said. "Can you come up to the kitchen?"

"Sure, I'll be there in a minute."

When I came up, there were a few residents in the kitchen along with Carol. He was placing what looked like a birthday cake on the table.

"This is for you.," he said.

"What? For me?"

"All the best Anna Maria" was written on it. Carol took a few pictures as everyone clapped and wished me well on my journey from Le Ricochet.

"You will be flying on your own now!" he said with such sincerity and emotion that it touched my heart.

Shortly after that, the secretary at Le Ricochet called and asked if I would write an article for the local newspaper for Mental Health Week. I was only too happy to do it, and it appeared a couple of weeks later along with one of the pictures Carol had taken on the day I left.

David knew I was looking for an apartment, so he was just as surprised as I was when Louise suddenly found this amazing place for me. When he came up to see it and met with Raymond and Suzanne, it was comforting to see how positive they were about my moving in. With that good interaction, I knew this was the best possible outcome.

After our brief conversation, Suzanne wanted to show us her beautiful flower garden, which she said was her passion.

"It requires a lot of time, but I love it," she said.

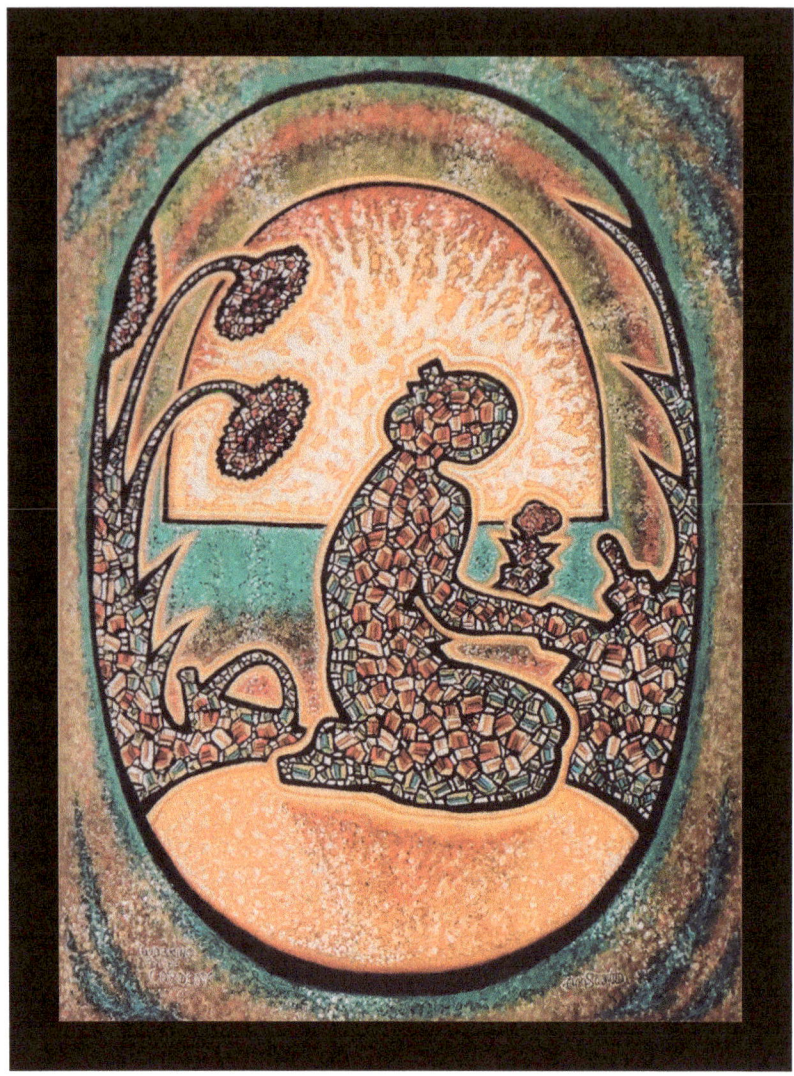

WORKING IN THE GARDEN

This inspired me to create my next expression, as the title popped into my mind right then and there: *Working in the Garden*. The image and title always comes into my mind first, followed by the actual creation itself. I wanted to begin as soon as I was settled into the apartment.

I had a really good sleep that first night just knowing that I could not have found a better place and that this all came about because of Louise Beauchemin's constant support. I was simply filled with gratitude.

The next morning, I was up bright and early. I got right into my routine of sitting in meditation and doing yoga exercises. I chose a spot in front of the large sliding glass doors that had an incredible view of the low-lying mountains. Their large, modern, light grey brick house partially sat on the side of the mountain. The sliding glass doors opened onto a cement patio that was sheltered from the neighbours houses. All I could see were the beautiful, tall spruce, pine, and maple trees.

After doing my spiritual practices in the morning and then spending time on my artwork, I would prepare a lunch. After my morning walk, I'd head over to Le Ricochet, which Louise said I was welcome to do whenever I felt like it. I found myself going over most days during the week. David was always with me on weekends; either I went to his place in Ottawa or he'd come up to Masham.

One morning while absorbed in my artwork, Raymond came creeping carefully down the stairs with an armful of food for the freezer.

"Elle travaille dur (She works hard)," he whispered.

They were always so considerate and polite, making me feel accepted and respected as an artist.

When I had completed *Working in the Garden*, Suzanne liked it so much she wanted to buy it. It was a side view of a woman kneeling down and planting flowers. I did it in what I called my "gemstone technique," and I mounted it with a velvet mat and gold frame. I must say it fit beautifully where she placed it on the wall in her dining room which opened up into a large glass solarium with a fantastic view of the surrounding hills. A perfect spot to simply enjoy the scenery or to just sit and read a book.

Satisfied with the completion of *Working in the Garden*, I felt ready to start on my next picture—the one I had put on the back burner until I knew for sure that David and I would be together. I eagerly immersed myself in this one, which I had already given the title *To Our Future Together*. Today, as I sit here writing, it is hanging on my bedroom wall alongside another one I titled *Flowers from My Love*, which I did after David gave me a beautiful bouquet of red roses. These two pieces are displayed as a set. I keep these memories alive through my art, expressing the special moments we shared in the beginning of our relationship.

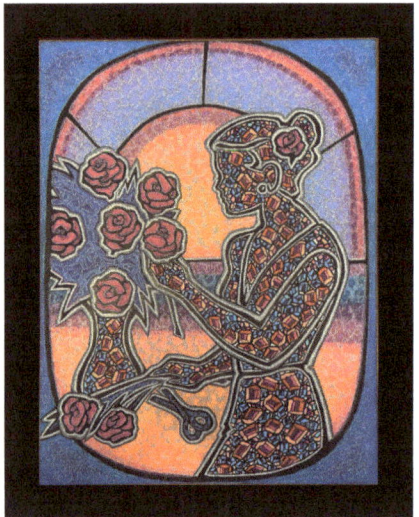
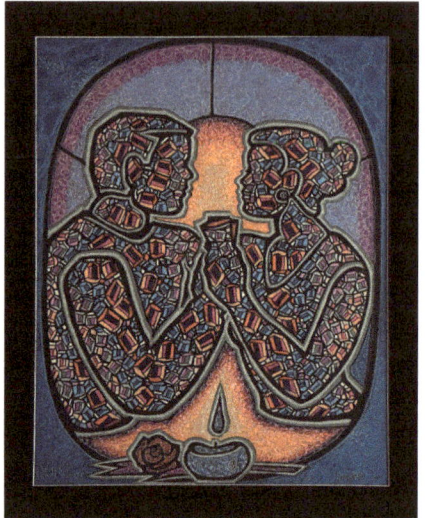

FLOWERS FROM MY LOVE

TO OUR FUTURE TOGETHER
Toasting to our future together on
Mothers Day - May 9th, 1999

As with every couple, there are always obstacles to overcome. With David and me, it was mainly dealing with my triggers. I'd hoped they would magically disappear once I found my soulmate, but even with the three years of therapy I had gratefully received while living at Le Ricochet, I still found myself struggling with them. They were always caused by a wrong perception where I thought I was not accepted or wanted.

David was like no other whenever I misunderstood something. He was always there with the patience of a saint to reassure me that this was not the case—that, in fact, I was accepted and wanted, and that he loved me very much. He never failed to bring me right back on track.

This kind of attention was totally new for me. I'd never had anyone make an effort like that to actually understand what was happening and why I had this wrong perception in the first place. He began to notice how quickly I recovered when he told me I was *not* being rejected or ignored. I was amazed how I was able to simply go on with my day as if nothing happened once I had that reassurance from him.

When I was living with Bruce, it often took me two to three days to get past the pain after experiencing a trigger. I am not blaming Bruce at all because he had no clue as to how to deal with someone like me. He was used to my sudden change in personality whenever I thought he didn't want to connect with me. But at that time, neither Bruce nor I realized that I had actually changed from Anna Maria to a personality I called "Deana." I am beginning to see now that I had been having these triggers not only with Bruce but with everyone else who I thought did not want to connect with me.

This was a real eye-opener for me, and I feel so sorry he had to live through that experience. I wish it never happened. In contrast, the immediate help I had from David right after experiencing a trigger made all the difference in the world. It was as if I was now being spared that mental and emotional aftermath.

Years after our divorce when I was living in Ottawa, Bruce said things might have turned out differently had he known what I went through after suffering those triggers. I doubt it, since we were very different on an emotional level. I needed someone with the capacity to understand me and to be there when I needed attention. I see now that I was unconsciously looking for my soulmate. I am thankful that David answered my ad and we had lunch on that very special Mother's Day in 1999; it really did change my life forever.

David said he began to observe abrupt changes in my personality whenever I'd have a wrong perception. After he pointed this out, we began to witness for ourselves how I instantly changed from Anna Maria to a different personality altogether. I began to call it my "other headspace." Gradually, as we became aware of what was happening during those moments, we were able to understand more. We discovered there was a pattern where I instantly switched from my friendly childlike personality of Anna Maria to a much stronger personality that was clearly being protective of her.

I actually named this personality Deana. She never failed to step in to protect Anna Maria, and I finally began to see why I had such a difficult time connecting with people all my life. It always confused me.

David mentioned that this was evident in the beginning of our relationship but he had no intention of giving up on me. Instead, he chose to stay, believing it was possible for us to have a good life together regardless of this unusual challenge. I began to come to terms with the fact that these triggers were not going to go away anytime soon, and I believed that with David by my side, there was still a chance to make a happy life for ourselves. I needed the support only David could give in addition to my spiritual practices that guide me on life's journey.

I vividly recall a moment back when I was living at the residence. Clair happened to be on duty, and I don't remember what we were talking about, but it was the first time anyone pointed out to me that I had this sudden switch in personalities. She was sitting on the couch in the living room when I approached to ask her a question. When she answered rather quickly and then stood up and said, "Oh, there's something I forgot to do," I immediately jumped to the conclusion that I must be bothering her. I suddenly had this wrong perception that she didn't want me there, and I blurted out, "Don't worry I won't bother you anymore!" and walked away in a huff.

She followed me into the kitchen and said, "Anna Maria, you CHANGED! What did I do to make you so upset?"

She moved away from me as if I was intimidating her. When I saw this, I composed myself and apologized.

"It's okay. I was just surprised about how you seemed so different all of a sudden, that's all," she said.

Later that night, I racked my brain trying to understand why I had behaved in such a way and promising myself this would never happen again. I am thankful that Clair and I continued to have a good relationship, but that incident made me aware of just how volatile my personality was.

With David's patience and understanding, we were able to delve deeper into what was going on inside my head that brought so much turmoil into my life for so many years.

One day, I received a phone call out of the blue.

"Hello, is that Anna?"

"Yes, speaking," I replied.

"Hi, this is Lynn. Your daughter."

I took a deep breath.

"Really? Lynn Marie? Oh my God!"

I was absolutely stunned.

She was only six weeks old when Dougie took her back to Cape Breton in 1965. I saw her only the one time after that when I flew down to Cape Breton and had to see them at school because Dougie wouldn't let me see any of my kids. So I was blown away when I heard Lynn Marie's voice on the phone. I could hardly believe it!

She said she would come to visit if I wanted to see her. She said that a girlfriend of hers who happened to be a soldier, would be passing through Ottawa on the way to her military base the next day. Could this really be happening? I was beside myself with excitement. She was patient and generous over the phone, filling me in without any hesitation or questions I had regarding her childhood in New Waterford.

She said she was living near Halifax and was happily married to a soldier. They had five children: four boys before finally having the girl they were hoping for; she was about two years old.

"I always wanted to have a large family," she said.

We arranged to meet the next day when her soldier friend brought her to Ottawa. She'd be staying for that long weekend. I called Robert in Montreal with the exciting news, and I was overjoyed when he said he would come to meet his sister for the first time.

"I should be there in a day or two," he said, "depending on the amount of work I have to do here."

When I turned into the gas station just outside Ottawa where we'd decided to meet up, I saw the car Lynn had described, so I slowly pulled up next to it. As I did, I recognized the soldier's uniform her friend was wearing. They were all smiles when they saw me.

As Lynn and I got out and happily embraced, she appeared as I had imagined. Her hair was similar to the picture I took that day of her and Elizabeth Anne at the school. She looked so cute with her bangs accentuating her high cheek bones, along with that overall clean, healthy look. I had always anticipated this day would come for us, but with the passage of time, along with her father's determination to keep us apart, I must admit I did have my doubts it would actually happen. But there we were! Despite the obstacles, my Ba Ba must have decided to finally reunite us.

I was extremely grateful to Lynn for initiating this meeting, since my attempts had always failed. We got into my car for the forty-minute drive to my place, and I realized she was tired from her long trip from Nova Scotia. So even though I was excited and wanted to know more about her and the grandchildren, I knew I should wait until tomorrow; there was so much I wanted to know about her life that I had missed, and vice versa.

Fortunately, my apartment had two large bedrooms, so she had her own room. We were having breakfast together the next morning when Robert called to say he was on his way and should arrive within a couple of hours. Meanwhile, Lynn and I settled down on the couch with an album of photos from the time I was living with Lee, Robert's biological father.

Both of us were happy and eager to know more about each other's past, but I misunderstood a comment she made about a photo of Lee. I took it as a criticism and immediately switched from Anna Maria to Deana, responding with a sharp, sarcastic remark. She suddenly recoiled with a look of surprise and confusion. Then stood up and calmly walked to the bedroom, closing the door behind her. I'd seen others act in a similar manner whenever Deana said something disparaging, but this was Lynn! How could this happen? I went to my room with a heavy heart, convinced I had ruined any chance of us getting to know each other.

Moments later, I realized I had changed back into Anna Maria, and I wanted to knock on her door to console her. But I suddenly became paralyzed with fear at the thought of being rejected by her. I began sobbing quietly into my pillow when I heard the doorbell ring. I knew it must be Robert, so I rushed to open it. His smile turned to a look of concern as he entered the apartment.

"What's wrong?" he asked.

I felt so ashamed that all I could say was that Lynn was in her room and that we had some kind of misunderstanding. That's when the bedroom door opened and Lynn slowly walked out with tears in her eyes. *This can't be happening!* I thought. Lynn turned to Robert with a look of sheer helplessness as she sat down at the table, motioning for him to sit next to her. My mind began racing with a terrible feeling that she didn't want me there.

Should I simply introduce them and then leave them alone?

I wasn't sure. It definitely was awkward for the three of us.

I timidly pulled out a chair and sat down next to Lynn. Robert seemed to understand immediately that I must have said something to upset Lynn. He wanted to help smooth things out, so he focused on her using a reassuring tone to make her feel welcome. I was so thankful because I was at a loss for words and honestly did not know how to handle the situation. After all, I was the mother and I should have been the one to solve this sticky situation I had brought about in the first place!

Realizing my own incompetence, I thought it would be better if I left them alone to connect. Robert would not be able to stay more than a few hours, so I started preparing lunch, hoping everything would be cleared up by then. I had confidence in Robert because he was always so calm. He was more rational than emotional, as I tend to be, so I felt he would do a better job communicating with her. It was interesting to see how similar Robert and Lynn were in terms of temperament, which gave me a sense that everything would soon be sorted out so that we could go on with our day amicably.

When I heard a sort of giggle from Lynn, I breathed a sigh of relief. *She must have gotten over our little incident*, I thought. It was heartwarming to see how happy they were to have finally met.

My main desire was to have a close, loving relationship with Lynn, but now I wasn't sure she felt the same way. It made me realize how poorly my mind had been functioning going right back to day one when I arrived on this planet. It dawned on me that the damage might not even be repairable.

I had been struggling for so many years, hoping somehow there would be a change so I could interact with others without having to worry about sudden triggers. I began to wonder if I should just distance myself from people again (as I did when I was living with Bruce). Otherwise, I felt I could continue to make an effort to connect but never know if or when some misunderstanding would cause everything to go awry. I was pretty tired of this emotional roller coaster, but I kept on believing I might eventually conquer this.

My recent connection with David had inspired me to move forward with confidence that I could handle anything that came my way, but this setback made me think twice. *Was I just fooling myself when I chose to believe I could actually have a so-called normal life? But how can I?* I asked myself, *if I'm always on edge when it comes to connecting with people, especially in social settings where I never felt comfortable.* And now this incident with my own daughter! Seeing how she reacted—like everyone else—was when I began to see the other person's side of the equation for the first time.

The three of us became quite comfortable with each other by lunchtime, though. We learned about each other's lives and talked about getting together in the future. After Robert headed back to Montreal, I asked Lynn if she'd like to come with me to Lac Philippe and was delighted when she showed some interest. By then I was convinced she had let go of any negative feelings towards me, and I became confident that if given time, we'd get to know each other better. I had to proceed with caution and be ever so careful to prevent any further incidents from happening, so I wasn't 100% comfortable.

As we walked along the beaches at Lac Philippe—there are three lovely sandy beaches—we rested at the picnic tables along the way as she shared information about herself, Andy and Elizabeth Anne. They were all in their thirties, and I wanted to know more about their lives.

I found out that Andy had never worked in the mines as his father did but took a welding course and ended up working in the oil sands at Fort McMurray, Alberta, on a seasonal basis. That's where many people from Cape Breton found good paying jobs as the mines had been closing down. She said Andy was married with two children, a boy and a girl, and his house was within walking distance from his father's on Roaches Road.

That's where Elizabeth Anne, known as Liz, had been living ever since Dougie and I separated in 1964. She had never married or had children. Lynn said Elizabeth Anne was a little slow in school, so I assumed there must have been some damage done to her brain that time she was turning blue and required oxygen right after she was born. I was not aware of any problems during that first year I had her with me, so it must have only become apparent after she started going to school. In retrospect, I can see that the best outcome for her was to have been brought up by the Campbell family, where she had a much more stable and secure environment than I could have provided for her in Montreal. So I took solace in the fact that all three of them were happy with the lives they had growing up in New Waterford and was grateful Lynn found me when she did.

I asked if she remembered when I came to see her at their school when she was six. She said yes and was interested in finding out more about that trip. I told her it was a short visit since things didn't work out as I had hoped, and that when I flew back home, I promised myself I would return to connect with the three of them the next time. That didn't actually happen until a few years later when I was married to Bruce.

"I became discouraged when Olga told me that none of you had any interest in seeing me," I said. "But as I was about to leave, I managed to get a hold of Andy on the phone. He was nineteen at that time, so I figured he had decided for himself when he agreed to meet with me at my sister Adeline's house on the outskirts of New Waterford. He was only two years old the last time I saw him, which was when we had that terrible car crash on our way back to Cape Breton."

When I finally spoke with Andy over the phone for the first time, he seemed quite distant, almost reluctant to meet with me. I more or less had to persuade him to come. He said he'd be there at a certain time but would wait outside. He didn't want to come into the house, which was just fine with me. *As long as I get to see him*, I thought. I was still hoping though that Elizabeth Anne and Lynn might show up with him, but that never happened.

Adeline and I were sitting in her living room near the large window and could see the car as it turned off the highway and began moving slowly towards the house. On impulse, I jumped up and rushed out the door. From the angle of vision I had while approaching the car on the driver's side, I saw the window winding down as I came up close. In my excitement,

I spontaneously burst out "ANDY!" To my surprise, the driver just sat there staring at me with this strange expression transfixed on his face as if he was somehow disappointed.

"No, I'm Andy," I heard from the passenger's seat.

Bending over to get a better look, I saw someone on the passenger's side, but he was slouched down as if not wanting to be seen.

"ANDY? Oh my God! I didn't see you! I'm terribly sorry!"

We were both at a loss for words, and it was clear that any interest he might have had to connect with me had vanished. He was humiliated in front of his friend and he changed his mind and just wanted to leave. I had never felt so embarrassed and ashamed in my entire life!

"Well that was a short visit!" said Adeline as I entered the house.

I went directly to a bedroom, threw myself onto the bed and burst into tears. She wanted to know what went wrong, but I was unable to speak about it. I asked if I could just be alone for a while.

An hour or so later, I explained the situation and asked if she'd drive me to the airport as soon as I could catch a flight back home. That futile attempt to see the three of them left me feeling terribly disappointed, but I was more concerned about Andy. It bothered me that I had put him in that embarrassing situation. I was the one who wanted to connect, and I felt somewhat remorseful for forcing him.

I spent most of the flight home ruminating about what took place and found myself becoming more distraught the more I thought about it. I was afraid it would be the last time we would see each other.

Lynn and I left Lac Philippe, and I was beginning to feel emotionally exhausted. I expended a lot of energy connecting with Lynn that day and it was a bit much. At the same time, it was quite therapeutic to express all the emotion I had experienced in those interactions.

Lynn seemed to be just fine, and she seemed more encouraged and satisfied as the day went on. I felt fortunate to spend that time with her, and David was happy to meet her before she left at the end of that long weekend. Her soldier friend, who was on her way back from the army base, took her back to Nova Scotia with her.

Driving back to my apartment after dropping Lynn off, I was so inspired by our time together that I was already considering the possibility of David and I making our own trip to Nova Scotia in the near future.

After Lynn arrived back in Nova Scotia, she arranged for a three-way telephone conversation with Liz. Andy got on the phone call, too, but he was still reserved. He basically answered yes or no to my questions, so I kept it short. But just the fact that he spoke to me again was enough, so I kept in touch with an occasional call to see how he was doing. Thankfully, Lynn and Liz were always open to communicating with me, so I stayed in touch with them.

Chapter 26

I had an unexpected call one day from Cheryl, one of the caregivers from Le Ricochet. We had kept in touch since I'd moved into Suzanne and Raymond's place two years before, but today's call was a surprise. She'd remembered my sixtieth birthday was coming up soon and wanted to invite David and I out for dinner at one of our favourite restaurants in nearby Wakefield.

It was quite a special day. I certainly did not feel like I was sixty, probably because I took good care of myself on all levels—physical, mental and spiritual—most of my life. Before leaving for the restaurant, Raymond and Suzanne came downstairs to share a piece of birthday cake with us, and when David and I arrived at the restaurant, Cheryl was there to greet me with a lovely bouquet of flowers. I was touched by her genuine effort to make me feel accepted. I don't know if she realized how much her attentiveness and concern for my well-being helped, not only when I was at the residence but afterwards as well.

A year later, the time had finally come for me to leave Raymond and Susanne's. Suzanne's family home, which was on their large property, was about to be renovated. Her mother was still living there but would stay in the basement apartment while the renovations were underway.

Had I wanted to live in Ottawa with David, I could, but he knew by now that, if given the choice, I would opt to live in the country. He was well aware of my reluctance to live in the city—any city. I had a deep underlying fear of being lost in a city, which was a psychological problem that had held me back from moving in with him. This aversion started back when Mama abandoned Anita and me in Montreal when we were seventeen.

I found an older farm house in a very quiet country setting near Rupert. I didn't know if I could handle living there alone, but I went ahead and took the apartment anyway, hoping I'd quickly adjust. I consciously threw myself into my art and tried to spend more time doing my spiritual practices, which were a priority in my day-to-day living. And I made sure I got out for long walks on the country roads regularly.

It was like living with Bruce, but I was completely alone. I never felt isolated at Suzanne and Raymond's since the door to the upstairs was always open, giving me a feeling of connection. So within a few weeks of moving into my new place, I began to wonder if I made the right decision. I tried to ignore the feeling of isolation, hoping I would soon get used to it, but that never happened. Whenever I'd entertain thoughts of moving to the city, I'd become overwhelmed with that terrible fear of being lost again. I wanted nothing more than to be with David because we loved each other and I missed him during the week.

Shortly after I took the apartment, I told David I would like to have a kitten to keep me company. He suggested I go online on his computer when I was in Ottawa the next weekend to find what I wanted. I had never used a computer before I met David, so not long after we started seeing each other he showed me how to send emails and some other basic things.

After checking out the different breeds of cats online, I chose a five-month-old female kitten from the "Munchkin" breed. The breeder was in Florida, which meant it would have to be flown up to Ottawa. The one that caught my eye was mostly black with white whiskers and paws and a white tuxedo marking on the chest. Compared to other cats, this breed is rather small; females were about 6 lb., males 8 lb. They have short legs and long bodies.

It was funny what happened once I had made my selection. I was asked if I wanted her spayed along with the required shots before sending her off to me. I replied yes in my email, but the next day I received a message from the vet that *she* turned out to be a *he*! They asked if I still wanted that cat.

I'd already fallen in love with this kitten from the photos, so gender was no longer important. I decided to name him Munchkin, after the breed. Arrangements were made to put him on a flight to Ottawa the next day.

I immediately noticed the difference it made having this little guy follow me around all day. I started to call him my little shadow. The character traits I read about him were right on, and I loved how sweet and affectionate he was right from the beginning. He helped keep me from feeling lonely during the week, and when David came up from Ottawa to be with me, Munchkin tried his best to distract us when we were sitting at the table talking. He'd walk towards the bathroom meowing loudly and wanting me to follow him. He made it clear that he did not want David around. It was so comical to watch his little mind trying to figure out how to get rid of him.

As time went on, though, I had to face the fact that living alone in the country was not working. After two years of resisting the temptation to live with David, something just snapped inside my brain one day. I hadn't planned it or even known it was going to happen. One Sunday night as David was getting ready to go back to Ottawa, I was suddenly overcome with this awful sinking feeling where I absolutely dreaded the thought of us being apart again. *Valentine's Day is next Tuesday, so why not just go back with him to Ottawa now? I thought.* It was like turning a switch inside my head where this feeling of sheer determination took over. I pulled my overnight bag out of the cupboard and said, "I've changed my mind. I'm not going to Ottawa on Tuesday as I said I would. I want to go now!" He was totally surprised and clearly quite happy with my spur-of-the-moment decision.

But he had no idea what was swirling around in my head.

That this was a pivotal moment in my life. I'd finally decided I would not allow this fear to control my life any longer! I decided right then and there that I would never spend another night alone in that apartment. David noticed I was acting a little strange as he helped to put Munchkin's carrier on the passenger seat next to me, but he didn't say anything. Just gave me a hug and a pat on the back. Then we hopped into our vehicles and headed to Ottawa where I had every intention of staying.

With each of us driving separately, there was no way to talk about what had just happened, so it had to wait until we got to David's place. When we arrived, he started winding down and preparing for his next day's work schedule. *On second thought,* I said to myself, *maybe I should wait until Monday to tell him. What if I were to suddenly change my mind?* I concluded it would be best to wait until Tuesday, Valentine's Day, as a surprise. I could hardly wait to tell him, but I also wanted to be absolutely sure this was the right move. David often wondered if and when I'd come to live with him permanently, so I was pretty sure he would be in favour of it.

I had been making the thirty-minute trip to Ottawa almost every second weekend with Munchkin beside me in his carrier, so he was used to being at David's by then. He was an indoor cat that was always at home except for when I took him to the vet or to David's. He liked to go downstairs to see David's mother who really enjoyed his company.

When Tuesday arrived, we had our little celebration. He gave me flowers, and we exchanged cards, as usual, before going out for dinner. I wanted so much to tell him about this dramatic shift, and I had to pinch myself to confirm that this transformation had actually taken place. We were having dinner at a vegetarian restaurant I loved called The Table, which was walking distance from David's place, when I finally felt it was time to let him know. *Well,* I thought, *I still have that same determination I had on Sunday, so I might as well tell him.* I wanted to know what he thought, and I needed to be sure I was making the right decision and that he really did want me to be there with him. I was taking a slight risk by proposing this major change, and I could have been setting myself up for a dreaded trigger.

It was a rather delicate, almost scary, position to put myself in. I couldn't help myself and went straight to the point.

"I know you were really surprised on Sunday when I suddenly wanted to come back to Ottawa with you," I said.

"Yes, I thought that was unusual because whenever you spend the weekend in the city with me, you always seem anxious to get back to the country. But I'm glad you're here with me now, so why not stay the rest of the week? Better still, stay over the weekend as well."

That response relieved any doubt I had about him wanting me there.

"David, you already know how much I wanted to be with you after I left Le Ricochet, but that crippling fear I had of living in the city always held me back. So today I want to tell you something truly extraordinary. As you were getting ready to leave my apartment on Sunday—I can hardly believe it myself—I suddenly refused to allow that fear to control my life any longer! A powerful tidal wave of certainty swept over me as I decided right then and there that this was the time for me to leave Rupert and spend the rest of my life with you where I truly belong."

David was listening intently as if amazed. Then he took my hand and gently pulled me up from my chair.

"Come on, give me a hug," he said. "Happy Valentine's Day, sweetie pie. You will always be safe with me here in Ottawa, so don't worry about the future; everything will work out just fine."

Needless to say, it was the most memorable Valentine's Day ever. My mind finally felt free to make other decisions that I may have backed away from had this not happened. Taking back my own power to make a life-changing decision such as this enabled me to move forward in my relationship with David. He turned out to not only be the soulmate I had been looking for but my guardian angel as well.

Shortly afterwards during my annual check-up with my family doctor in Wakefield, I mentioned my impending move and wanted to know if I could be referred to a doctor at the Royal Ottawa, a psychiatric hospital. I assumed that since our prime minister's mother, Margaret Trudeau, had been a patient there, they must have the best of care.

When I showed up for my appointment with Dr. Kraus, I discovered they were not able to take me as a patient because I did not, in fact, have bipolar disorder after all. Here's what the notes I have on file say:

> Thank you for referring this very interesting and challenging woman to the Mood Disorders Program at the Royal Ottawa Hospital. Your referral note indicated a past diagnosis of bipolar disorder, but she has never actually been psychiatrically hospitalized, and has been on no psychotropic agents for a number of years. She describes chronic life long difficulties which are not much different now than they ever have been. Her symptoms include intense abruptly changing mood swings, and always in reaction to a trigger of some sort of an interpersonal nature. Typically this is something involving either perceived criticism, or perceived rejection.
>
> It was actually quite interesting at the very end of today's interview when she demonstrated this exact process with me, suddenly becoming very cold, sullen, and clearly angry at me, announcing "You don't like me very much, do you?" when nothing was further from the truth. This seemed to be in direct reaction to my trying to explain to her that we did not have the resources here to help her, and when I was trying to suggest some other possibilities: a setup for perceived rejection, she obviously took this as criticism and was seemingly angry in response.
>
> This woman's lifelong description of difficulties including recent symptoms, and her pattern of interacting within this interview are almost certainly reflective of "borderline personality" and not reflective of bipolar disorder, or any other primary mood disorder. Patients with borderline personality disorder have all the aforementioned features that she suffers from, especially interpersonal difficulties. The treatment of choice should be community based long

term psychotherapy, and not hospital-based psychiatric services. Pharmacotherapy has very little or no place in the management of such patients, especially in someone like her who has never had a psychiatric hospitalization in the past.

So I had been misdiagnosed years ago. Unfortunately, my appointment with the second doctor that he had referred me to ended with me walking out, so I realize now that I should have found another doctor, but I didn't.

Somewhere along the way it dawned on me, that in our society when one suffers from a physical ailment - it is accepted. But not so when one suffers from a mental condition, that there definitely is a stigma attached - making it much more difficult for one to cope.

It may appear that my decision to go to Ottawa was only because I couldn't stand the isolation any longer. It was a major factor but definitely not the only one. In fact, deep down I had always wanted to be with David and I'm sure he knew this.

After making the choice to stay in Ottawa with David, I had to learn to find my way around the city by car when David was not with me. I did pretty well when I used to travel because I wrote down the major routes and found my way from city to city, but now when it came to simply shopping not far from David's house, it was a different story. I'd find my way to the shopping malls all right, but as I was about to exit the parking lot, I'd forget which direction I should turn. *Do I turn right? Or left?* Only after I had driven some distance did I realize I was going in the wrong direction, so there I was in the flow of traffic searching for a place to turn around. I'd frantically grab my phone and call David.

"David! I'm sorry to bother you but I'm lost! I'm at the corner of [such and such a street]. Can you please tell me where to go from here?"

Of course, he'd always take a few minutes to guide me back to where I had lost track.

It doesn't sound like much, but in the beginning when it happened, I was in tears and he'd have to take a few moments to calm me down. For quite some time after that, I'd have incredible anxiety attacks whenever I'd get into my car to go shopping. It was like some kind of victory every time I'd go and come back without any problem.

Eventually I became so familiar with driving in Ottawa that the stress disappeared. I became comfortable not only with driving in the city but living there as well. I can't imagine living anywhere else now. I love being surrounded by all the conveniences the city has to offer.

Chapter 27

I had been living with David for about a year when I reconnected with an agency at the hospital in Montreal where Steven was born and where I had to give him up for adoption when he was only five days old. I had been in touch with them off and on over the years as they tried to find Steven for me, but they never had any luck.

When I called to give them my new telephone number at David's place, I was surprised when they told me they had recently found Steven's adoptive parents. The only information they had was he had been adopted into a family who lived in the United States, and I was given a telephone number to call.

I phoned and spoke with his adoptive mother, a nice lady who gave me basic information before I was able to speak with him. She said they had raised Steven in the Cape Cod area, not far from Boston. When he became an adult, she said he wanted to go to Brazil, where he was now living and working as a Bible teacher.

A few days later, I received a call from Steven. He had recently married and his wife was pregnant with their first child. He also said he had plans to come to Canada, but they were having troubles getting her into Canada legally. I don't remember the whole story as I was more caught up in what was happening on the emotional level.

We finally met Steven when he came to David's place by himself; his wife was still in Brazil. They wanted their baby to be born in Canada, so they were trying to figure out how to do that. Robert and David had been waiting with me in great anticipation on the day he was to arrive when the doorbell rang.

"That must be Steven!" I said as I rushed down the stairs to meet him in the vestibule.

When I opened the door, he smiled and stepped inside as Robert and I greeted him with a gentle hug. I nervously reached for my camera to get a photo, then he followed Robert and I upstairs to where David was waiting patiently. He seemed cautious, so I quickly composed myself and tried not to overwhelm him as I had a tendency to do when excited.

It was the Christmas season because the tree was still up. We made him feel comfortable as we welcomed him with open arms and shared his concern about his wife coming to Canada as soon as possible. I could hardly believe he was actually there with us! I was looking forward to getting to know about his life, and I was so thankful he had been adopted into the loving home I had prayed for when I gave him up for adoption.

David was happy to show him around our area when he expressed a desire to find a place to rent here in Ottawa, and he wanted to help in any way he could. A couple of days later when we were a little more relaxed with each other, the subject of religion came up. He mentioned he was a Bible teacher in Brazil, and I was happy that he had found his vocation. I mentioned I had been on this spiritual path for many years and how much I had benefitted from it. To my dismay, his demeanour suddenly changed and he became quite serious—almost as if he didn't approve. I immediately understood where he was coming from because of my strict religious background; I knew just how inflexible the thinking can be sometimes.

"Maybe we'll have to be careful so that our beliefs don't divide us rather than unite us," I said respectfully.

I thought this cautionary note might help, but instead it made him uncomfortable and he quickly changed the subject to his immediate concern about getting his pregnant wife to Canada as soon as possible. I was very uneasy after that, thinking I must have been too direct. *Maybe I shouldn't have said anything at all*, I thought.

He was clearly avoiding me the next day and only showed interest in speaking with David or Robert. I went to David's office where he had spent most of his time on the computer connecting with his wife in Brazil. I was startled when he quickly got up and pulled the door over slightly when he saw me coming.

"Sorry, but I need my privacy," he said in a serious tone.

I backed off immediately, not sure what to say or do. It was hard to shake off the feeling that this could be a stumbling block in our relationship. When it became obvious that he was not about to open his mind to accept my chosen path, I felt as if I was standing on the sidelines watching; we seemed to be drifting apart and I didn't know how to handle it.

Robert tried to console me by saying he understood my position, which helped. David also realized this was happening, but he, like Robert, seemed to think I should simply accept this outcome since there was nothing I could do about it. Steven left a few days later when he found a place he said he wanted to rent. He had been under great pressure to deal with getting his wife into Canada, so I couldn't help but feel empathy for him. It was more important than my little concern at the time.

However, I knew how the human mind can become conditioned when it comes to one's religion without realizing it. After giving it some thought, I concluded that he thought I was on the wrong path (like Mama used to think). I knew I'd likely be wasting my time if I tried to get him to accept the fact that there are more paths than one and that it would be much better if we were to simply accept and respect each other's chosen path.

Unfortunately it didn't turn out that way for us.

Sadly, after that visit we didn't hear anything more about him, his wife or even where they were living, so we have no idea where he is. I have often wondered how our lives might have turned out if only we could have come together as children of the Supreme rather than splitting apart as we did. There's still a glimmer of hope that somehow our paths might cross again someday; we never know what the future holds for any of us.

A few months after I moved to Ottawa, the warm weather finally arrived and I began to yearn for that fresh country air, along with the peace and quiet of my beloved Lac Philippe. David must have been aware that this longing for the country was tugging at me because he suggested we take a drive up there as soon as there was a nice sunny day.

"Do you think we could drop by Le Ricochet for a short visit?" I asked. "Since it's only minutes away from Lac Philippe?"

"Why not? Maybe you'll get to see Cheryl while we're there."

The following Sunday turned out to be a gorgeous day for such a trip, and when we stopped by, both Cheryl and Julie happened to be working. After a chat with them, we walked around to the back of the residence where David used to park when I lived there. As I was about to get into the car, I cheerfully waved hello to the neighbour.

"Who's that?" David asked.

"That's Robin. He has an excavation business there at home. He speaks English and is a nice friendly guy."

"Looks like he's having his land surveyed," said David. "See the tripod near the fence? If you don't mind, I'd like to go over and talk to him for a minute."

"Sure, go ahead."

A couple of minutes later he was back with a business card in his hand.

"Well, it's just as I thought," he said. "He's having his property surveyed to have it divided up into lots."

"Really? Are you interested in buying a lot from him?" I asked.

"It depends on how much he's charging; it just might be worth looking into."

"Well, this is an unexpected connection for sure," I said.

"I'm pretty sure my brother Stephen who is an architect could draw up some plans for a bungalow if I were to give him a general idea of what I'd like."

"You mean you'd be open to driving the half hour to Ottawa to get to work?"

"This Gatineau auto route is a breeze compared to the hour and a half I used to drive to get to work years ago, so that wouldn't be a problem. But first I'd like to find out the cost and whether or not it would be feasible."

This idea had popped up of out of nowhere, taking me by complete surprise.

"I'd better not get my hopes up too high about this," I said to David.

"Right, if it's not in our ballpark, then we'll have to let it go. But first we'll get more information before making any decisions, okay?"

It was almost noon, so we stopped to pick up poutine—French fries with little chunks of cheese smothered in gravy—from the stand near the corner. We rarely ate it, but that day we decided to go for it. What a lovely day that turned out to be. We were looking forward to a bright future, whether it be there in Masham or in Ottawa. It didn't matter all that much to me now. I was happy we were together and I knew the feeling was mutual.

David and I went downstairs to his mother's place to have dinner a few weeks later, as we often did on Sunday evenings. Mitzi had arrived with her boyfriend Del, who brought a bouquet of roses and placed them on the table. Mitzi brought a casserole that she made, and David and I put together a big salad. Alexis, who sometimes joined us for dinner, was at his mother's place that evening.

Whenever we got together at his mother's place, she always seemed to be open to having conversation while enjoying the attention she had from everyone. But that evening she appeared to be in a slightly different mood, and I remember near the end of the meal, Mitzi, who is quite jovial at times, raised her glass of wine saying, "Well, mother, here's to your hundredth!"

"Oh no! Don't wish that on me!" she said.

We all laughed. But David and I noticed she had left most of the food on her plate and was abnormally quiet. She then decided she wanted to leave the table.

"My stomach doesn't feel good," she said. "I think I'll lie down for a while."

So Mitzi helped her get ready for bed while we cleaned up in the kitchen.

Over the next week, Flo's health slowly deteriorated to the point where they thought they should call their minister to come and pray with the family as they were gathered around her bed. Flo had already decided she should be brought to a place called Maycourt, which was nearby. Her husband Ted had designed the palliative care unit there.

"Everybody wants to go there," she said.

When they took her to Maycourt a few days later, she was heavily sedated because of the pain. Mitzi had been by her side constantly as Flo drifted in and out of consciousness for close to a week. She was only weeks away from her ninety-ninth birthday when she finally did pass. Mitzi got the call at three o'clock in the morning telling her that Flo had passed peacefully during the night. It was November 23, 2008.

It was at a time when there was a high demand for real estate in their area, so David had to make a decision as to what to do with the duplex after his mother passed. It was right next to Fisher Park, where David used to water the rink for the kids to go skating during the winter and they played soccer during the summer. There was a large tennis court behind his place next to the park as well. It was amazing how quickly their duplex was sold. The For Sale sign was up only one day when it was bought.

Meantime, David found us a place only six minutes away in a nice apartment complex called Sawville Apartments. The three buildings, each one seven stories, had a large outdoor pool in its courtyard surrounded by beautiful trees. It also had another large, heated indoor pool, both of which had been upgraded with the switch from chlorine in the water to salt. It was just behind the Carlingwood Shopping Centre in the lovely suburban neighbourhood of Napean, so it was a perfect choice for us. And the four-minute drive to David's work turned out to be a real advantage.

While in the process of moving from his duplex to the Saville Apartments, David and I were clearing out his office when he called my attention to a large envelope he had in his hand.

"Remember that property I wanted to buy from Robin?" he asked.

"Yes, of course" I said.

"Well, these papers show his land had been surveyed at the time he gave property to his children. I was told it had to be surveyed again when he wanted to divide the rest up into lots to sell, like the one I was interested in a while back. Remember when our plan had to be put on hold because they were not available at the time I was interested?"

"Yes! Wow, things have really changed since I came to live here in Ottawa, eh Lovie?"

"They sure did—and for the better, I might add," said David.

"Aw, you always say such nice things," I said.

"Well, I'm thinking we've done enough here for today," he said. "Would you like to have some Chinese food for a change?"

"That sounds great! I know you really like the egg rolls from the Golden Palace, so maybe you'll order some along with a couple of vegetarian spring rolls for me?"

"You just read my mind, Sweetie Pie!"

It was January 2009 when David and I moved into the Saville Apartments. The walls had been painted an off-white, so I spent the next few weeks painting some of them in colours I preferred. I finally had our furniture nicely arranged to our satisfaction.

Having done all that, my mind turned to a trip to Cape Breton we had wanted to make a while back. David had an RV service business in the past, so he had lots of experience in that department and thought we should do the trip in an RV. So he went out and bought a new travel trailer. He took September off so we'd have enough time to get around to visit everyone.

The plan was for us to stop near Halifax at Lynn's house first to meet her husband and five children. He was stationed there at the time. We had booked for one night at a campsite on the way, but just before we got there, I saw in the outside mirror on my right some black pieces of material fly away from the trailer, but we didn't feel or hear anything.

"WOW, what was THAT?!"

"We may have blown a tire" he said calmly- I'll stop and check.

Shortly after a quick change of the tire, we reached the campsite where we were to spend the night.

When we arrived at Lynn's house the next day, I was happy and so excited to see her again and to meet her family. David parked the trailer in their long driveway where we were to park for the next few days and visit.

Munchkin seemed content in the trailer all the time, which made it easy for us since he didn't have that urge to explore outside. He was happy just looking out the window from the perch he had on the back of the couch.

When Lynn's husband John came in dressed in his army uniform, he appeared quite proud as he introduced himself in a rather reserved but cordial manner. After a brief conversation, he excused himself saying he had something to attend to. Just then the phone rang. Lynn answered, and when she hung up she said Liz was on her way from Cape Breton.

"But Andy is not coming," she said, "so his wife Donna is driving Liz over instead. Their daughter Brittany is with them. It'll be a few hours before they get here because they're coming from New Waterford."

When they arrived, I had my camera ready when Liz came through the door, followed by Donna and Brittany.

"What beautiful eyes," I said as I snapped a close-up of Liz.

"They're like yours," she said, as we gave each other a hug.

It was wonderful to have Lynn and Liz together. It was like a dream come true. I learned quite a bit about Lynn when she visited me in Masham, but I didn't know much about Liz, so I was happy to have this chance to spend time with her and get to know more about her life in New Waterford. Andy's absence, of course, left a gap, but I still had hope we would eventually get together—the light of hope was still burning.

The kids wanted us to go with them to the garage, where they showed us their two beautiful black and white rabbits. It was a pleasure to meet Lynn's children, starting with Mathew, the oldest, then Ethan, Adam, Jonathan and Rebeca. They seemed curious to meet us, but they were soon occupied with their own interests. In the evenings we sat outside in the backyard in their large gazebo where we had a lovely, expansive view of the fields and trees.

But all too soon the time had come to move on to our next stop. I appreciated that special time with everyone, and the pictures I took keep those memories alive as time marches on.

Our plan was to visit Anita and Howard next in Louisbourg, Cape Breton, where they had been living for a number of years. Their house was on a slight hill, and David had to carefully back up the trailer along their driveway. We found them sitting outside in the backyard looking quite cozy in front of a nice little fire they had made that was surrounded by bricks. I had never met Howard, and as we introduced ourselves, I instantly sensed he was a gentle soul, quiet and unassuming. They invited us to join them by the fire where we had a nice long chat before going into the house.

Anita was quite proud to show us her artwork that completely covered a whole wall in their living room. I was impressed with the number of oil paintings she had created of lovely scenes from around the area. She said she'd done pretty well with sales during the tourist season, as she always had a few on display in the gallery there. Anita and Howard both appeared to be quite content living in Louisbourg, and I was really happy for them. I gave her one of my own expressions as a souvenir, as I did when I visited Lynn.

The next day we had a little tour of the Louisbourg Fortress and had lunch afterwards at their place before starting out for Adeline's place in River Ryan, on the highway just outside of New Waterford.

When we turned into her driveway, I flashed back to that day Andy came to see me at her place. But my mind quickly bounced back as Adeline approached and I introduced her to David. He was quite interested in their large, dome-shaped garage with two large tractors inside. She mentioned it was her husband's business before he passed away a few years ago, and their son Wilfred was running it and she did the books.

Later that day, Wilfred dropped by with Charlotte, Adeline's daughter, who was a school teacher. Before we knew it, they were engaged in interesting conversation with David. He always had many interesting things to talk about, especially when we were in social situations. Since the attention was mainly focused on him, it helped to reduce the anxiety I was experiencing.

The next day, I told David I wanted to go in town because I wanted him to see a few places and meet some people.

"Okay, I will disconnect the trailer before we leave to make it easier for us to get around," he said.

The first place I wanted to show David was the house on Mahon Street where Anita and I were born and had lived until we were fifteen. As we pulled up in front, I was struck by the change that had taken place right next to the house itself. They had constructed a road, which now had row houses, where the large outdoor rink used to be between Mahon Street and St. Anne. David remained in the truck when I said I was going to knock on the front door to see what happened. The gentleman who opened the door showed interest when I told him I was born in that house back in 1942. His wife happened to be there with him and asked if I'd like to have a little tour, which was exactly what I had been hoping for.

We started downstairs where the big grey furnace that always had a huge load of coal next to it was gone. The basement had been turned into a rec room. The shiny coloured bricks that used to be around the fireplace in the living room had been replaced with plain, sand-coloured bricks, but the French doors were still there.

Upstairs in what used to be Mama and Papa's bedroom was now an office. One wall had been removed and a counter divided the room. Even with the changes that were made, my mind still held the images of how it used to be when I was a child.

They told me they bought the house from Justine and George after their adopted son moved out west. It was now owned by the son of the doctor who just happened to be my physician when I was pregnant with Andy back in 1962. They came outside to meet David, and as we were walking towards the truck, I pointed out that there used to be a large veranda across the front of the house with a wide, thick railing. He turned to his wife and said, "See! I figured there must have been something like that because of the large cement blocks we found buried there." When I asked about the new construction in the back, he said they were apartments for senior citizens who are still able to take care of themselves. George's mother sold their little bungalow across the street after his father died, moved into one of those units and really liked living there.

I thanked them for allowing me to have those moments of reflection and was grateful for their genuine hospitality. David was skeptical at first, but when he saw how well that little visit turned out, he was happy for me.

From there, we continued on to Plummer Avenue where Papa had his business many years ago. I was pleasantly surprised when I saw a huge, colourful mural that had been erected in the little park close to where our store used to be. It showed all the storefronts as they used to be along Plummer Avenue back in the 1930s and '40's, some of which were still there, and we could see exactly where our store was situated.

As we passed by the park where the statue stood in memory of the miners who lost their lives, I couldn't help but recall that day when I first saw Dougie pass by on his white horse. It was wonderful to go down memory lane with David by my side that day because I didn't get the chance to do that on my previous trips.

I wanted to drive along Roaches Road where Dougie and his family lived and where Andy, Liz and Lynn had been raised. As we drove slowly past their house, everything appeared different compared to when I lived there for that short time. Dougie's mother's house had been done over with a light beige siding, and I saw two racehorses outside near the barn.

I wanted to see that little bungalow where we lived without the bathroom. As we came to a stop in front the house, the first thing I noticed was it had been painted another colour and the outhouse that used to be in the backyard was gone. There was now a lawn with a fence across the front where the half-finished trench used to be.

The memories started to come back one after another, but it was strange because it felt as if everything that had taken place there had happened in another lifetime altogether. With David next to me, I was safe and secure, and I felt truly fortunate.

The fact that Liz, Lynn and Andy grew up in a stable environment with the Campbells on Roaches Road made me feel grateful beyond measure. God only knows what would have happened if they had remained in my care during that time of incredible struggle.

The experience of going back that day must have given me some kind of closure because I felt more at peace with myself afterwards. I must have let go of the shame and guilt I had been carrying around with me all that time.

After we got back to Adeline's place, I wanted to be alone for a while to sort out a number of things in my head. All the questions that lingered in my mind over the years had been answered, and aside from the fact that Andy didn't come this time, the connections I had made with Liz and Lynn seemed to have made up for it. I still had hopes of being with all my children one day—what is that expression? Hope springs eternal?

Shortly after I moved in with David, we were coming back from getting our groceries. He was about to turn into his lane when my white Toyota I had left parked in front of his garage began to move. It was backing up very slowly at the same time as David was turning into his driveway.

"What the heck?" David exclaimed, staring in disbelief.

"Someone's taking my car!" I said.

Whoever was behind the wheel slammed on the brakes and we almost ran into each other.

"Stay here!" David said, rushing over to see who was in the driver's seat. "What do you think you're dong?" he said angrily as he opened the door.

I was shocked to see it was ALEXIS! He slowly stepped out as his friend jumped out from the passenger's side. We'd arrived just before they left with my car! Evidently Alexis, having recently passed his driver's licence test was tempted when he saw my keys sitting on the kitchen cupboard. I don't know whether his friend had any influence over him or not, but apparently he decided to take my car for a spin before we returned with the groceries that day.

I didn't know what to think after that. I already felt he hadn't accepted me from day one, and in a way, I understood; he may have thought I was going to take his father away. But it had been a few years and he still remained distant with me. He never made eye contact or spoke to me. I kept thinking maybe he'd come around, but I had to accept the facts as they were presented there in front of me.

So I told myself to just let it go. The most important thing was to focus on my relationship with David, so I tried not to mention that little incident again. Aside from that, it was obvious David and had a good relationship, and I was not about to intervene. It took some time before he was able to accept me as his father's partner, although at arm's length, I would say. He remarked one time that he thought I made his father happy. This may be one of the reasons he stopped shunning me.

As we drove through New Waterford, I thought about Anita and how we had lost track of each other after spending almost thirty years living in Saint-Jean-de-Matha. After the children grew up and left the nest, Anita and I eventually left, too, as our relationships with Bruce and Jim had slowly deteriorated. Even then, we both still hoped to find lasting relationships. Anita met George, but, sadly, he became ill and passed away a couple of years after they were married. Eventually she met someone else when she was living in the little tourist town of Rawdon, just north of Montreal, where she was a member of the Artist's Circle. Even though she seemed to be doing okay, she told me she'd wanted to return to Cape Breton ever since Mama dropped us in Montreal. She finally decided to sell her little bungalow in Rawdon and move back to Cape Breton because she missed living near the ocean that she loved so much. I was never interested in returning to Cape Breton myself, and I only went back when I simply could not handle living in the city any longer.

Looking back, I find it interesting that even though Anita and I have the same background and carry similar mental and emotional scars, we ended up with different mental disorders. She mentioned she had been seeing a psychologist and was on medication for depression. The psychologist said hers was a case of severe mental and emotional neglect in childhood. No wonder we turned out the way we did. Carrying all that baggage made it difficult to move forward, especially when the future looked so bleak at times.

I find it fascinating just how similar our karma had been over the years. It started right from the beginning when we were rejected at birth, struggling to keep our babies, facing various traumas and situations that most people would never have experienced in their lifetime. Just the fact that we happened to be pregnant at the same time is unusual. I can't help but be amazed that despite the challenges, not only did we find the lasting relationships we had sought, but we are both living in places that we truly love.

Anita continues to paint beautiful pictures there on the east coast while I went from expressing emotion through my art to using words to describe the images for you to see in your mind. I must admit, though, that having no education to rely on made writing this book quite a challenge. Come to think of it, I've done everything without any academic training. Guess you'd say I am self-taught in that whatever I happened to be drawn to; I simply took it up on my own. Like art and drumming, for instance. Until David came into my life, I had never used a computer, but it didn't take me long to learn the basics. I'm not on social media or anything like that; I use it mainly for connecting by email and to Skype occasionally with Robert and his two little girls Milie and Daphnee.

When I first mentioned to Anita that I had started to write a book but wasn't sure whether or not it was book material, she wasn't interested. Others weren't either, so I definitely had moments of self-doubt as to whether or not I should continue. When I told her the title, it instantly brought back the memory of when Mama shook the poker at us saying "should've died when you were born! because she surprised me with- "Like the time she chased me with the knife."

"What? What do you mean?" I asked.

"Oh, I didn't tell you about that? Well, one time when I wanted to go outside but Mama wouldn't let me, I must have pestered a bit, because she suddenly grabbed a knife and chased me upstairs. I ran into the bathroom and locked the door. I was so scared I opened the window and crawled out onto the roof below."

"Wow, I didn't know about that, Anita! I'm surprised, but in a way, I'm not, since there were so many incidents like that over the years; you can't remember them all."

"Well, I certainly didn't forget that one! So when will the book be finished?" she asked.

"I have no idea since I've never attempted anything like this before. When you read it, I hope you won't be too upset with me for being so blunt in describing the struggles we've encountered. It's the only way I know how to do this. I need to express whatever it is I want to say exactly as I see it in my mind. I couldn't have been more transparent when exposing my own vulnerabilities and stupid mistakes. I didn't sugar-coat anything, it just wouldn't be me. But to be honest, I do have some concern about how others I've written about will react."

As we ended our phone conversation, I was feeling slightly uncomfortable because I didn't know what to expect. It's a given that I'd have to face the consequences should there be any repercussions down the road, but I know I will always have my Deana personality to rely on if needed. She has stepped in to protect my vulnerable personality, Anna Maria, ever since I can remember. As for the devotee Amrta personality—the artist who has been telling this story—she just might need a little support down the road. That's where Deana will have to come in as well. I must say, she has come a long way over the years in ascertaining just how to deal with conflict. So I am quite confident she will handle any problematic situation that might occur by being extra careful to approach it in a tactful manner.

Writing keeps my mind focused, as did my artwork, and I find it's all I want to do lately. As I move through my regular routine each morning, it takes a couple of hours before I even get started on the writing. I can't wait to get back to where I left off, to do some editing and create my next paragraph.

When we returned home after our trip to Cape Breton, David put his trailer into storage for the coming winter and was once again busy with his work at the condominium. He can control the operating facilities in the building from home on his computer, making it possible for us to have each other's company more often, which I like. I always preferred being at home because I was able to have that control of setting my own priorities while organizing my time to get everything done as I had wanted. I think this structured life I made for myself was necessary to keep me grounded. Even so, I still suffer from triggers every now and then. But compared to years earlier, my life is much better now—even somewhat normal.

It's been three years since I began writing this manuscript, and I can see how much my mind has changed over that period of time. Especially when it comes to my feelings about Mama and how we were raised without any nurturing or love from her whatsoever. Somewhere along the line, I realized the anger I was carrying around had actually stemmed from not being accepted at birth, so I finally managed to let it go and replace it with forgiveness. In doing so, I noticed I even had a bit of empathy for her, which I didn't expect. So with this change in thinking, I was able to move forward in the healing process and understand the meaning of unconditional love for the first time. It turned out to be a significant milestone in my life.

David's example played a huge part in helping me because he demonstrated what it was all about right from the beginning of our relationship. It took me a while I admit, but over time I was able to learn its true meaning from him. Consequently, I no longer blame myself for my past experiences, and I realize that there was bound to be some psychological scars as a result of the traumas I experienced. So I am much easier on myself lately, and I find I'm not as concerned as I once was with how I'm connecting with others. I have reached the point where I can honestly say that I feel free to just *be me*!

Talking about connections, one important one happened when I least expected it, and it was a wonderful surprise indeed. I was at home being the busy bee I usually am when Andy called. I was flabbergasted. He was the last person I anticipated hearing from, and I was thrilled to hear he'd had a change of heart and wanted to see me. He never had much to say the few times I did speak to him, so I kind of expected it when he kept it short and to the point.

"I'm on my way home from Fort McMurray and can pass through Ottawa and stop by for a short visit," he said.

I could hardly believe it.

"That would be wonderful, Andy! I'm so glad you called, and I can't wait to see you!"

I quickly put together a little snack and called David to tell him the good news. Minutes later, my phone rang.

"It's Andy, I'm downstairs.

"Great! I'll buzz you in. Do you have my apartment number?"

"Yes, I have it," he said.

I was a bit nervous as I waited for the elevator door to open, and I saw he, too, was a little unsure of himself as he stepped out. I immediately reassured him with a comforting hug.

"So when did you leave Fort McMurray?" I asked as we entered our apartment.

"Four days ago, sleeping in hotels along the way. I still have fourteen hours of driving to do before I reach New Waterford."

"Wow, that is such a long trip! I can't tell you how much this means to me, Andy."

"I can't stay very long, though; I really do have to get back on the road."

"Of course, I understand," I said as I led him outside onto the balcony.

He settled for a cold drink instead of the snack. It was a bright, sunny day, and I was really thankful that we were finally able to connect properly. I learned a bit about his life in New Waterford and his work out west before David suddenly popped in. He said he wanted to come and meet Andy while he had the chance. Andy was proud to show us videos he had recently taken at the harness races back home, where their horses were doing well, as always. But all too soon he said he had to be on his way, so I accompanied him down to his truck and reluctantly said goodbye.

As he pulled away, I immediately consoled myself that next time I would see all three of them—Andy, Liz and Lynn—together at the same time. So far, I've met Andy's wife Donna and daughter Brittany, but I have yet to meet his son Andrew.

Chapter 28

I started to feel the need to be among spiritual aspirants once again, so I got my computer out and found a spiritual centre close to us called the Ottawa Spiritual Pathways Centre (OSPC). It turned out to be in the Mason's heritage building where David's father used to be a member many years ago. The spiritual group renting space there was multifaith, which I was very comfortable with, and I really enjoyed the vibration there when we all sang their lovely songs together.

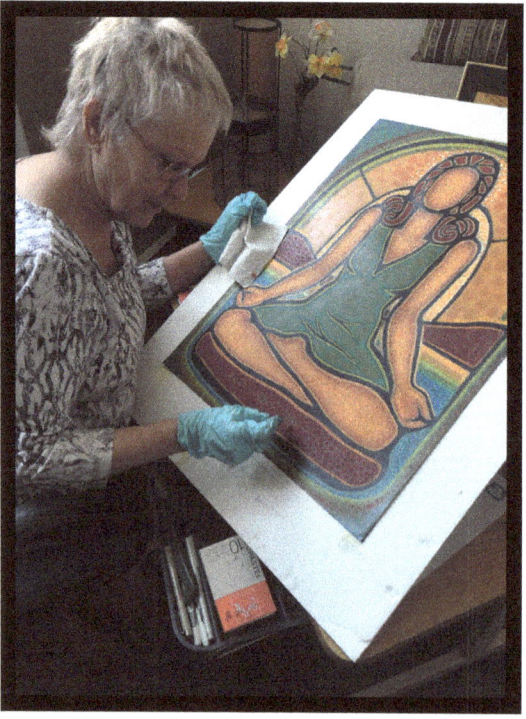

Anna Maria working on one of her creations

When I came home and shared my experience with David, he was rather curious, and after asking a few questions, he said he'd like to come with me the next time. I was delighted when he showed some interest since he had never done so before. After listening to the sermon and sharing in the music, I observed he had become quite comfortable, and before I knew it, we were attending the services together on a regular basis. This was in the spring of 2016.

We really liked the ambience at OSPC, and one Sunday as I was chatting with Rev. Nicole during fellowship time after the service, she asked if I would be interested in sharing a prayer or something during one of their services. I declined, of course, having never done anything like that before, but then found myself offering to bring my djembe African drum to play along to their lovely songs. *At least I could contribute in this way,* I thought. She agreed, and it was the beginning of sharing in their music. I was only too happy to be part of it because it had been quite a while since I had played for our akhanda kirrtans. I felt this was exactly what I needed at that time, and having David there with me made it that much more special.

The centre had been opened by Rev. Nicole and another spiritual aspirant two years prior to our joining. I was impressed when she told me she and her husband drove from Montreal to Ottawa every Sunday morning, a two-hour drive each way, in order to hold their service. And I must say I found it interesting how the timing had coincided with an unexpected phone call.

"Hello, Amrta? It's dada Sarvabodhananda, remember me?"

"Well, of course, dada. I recognized your voice right away, what a surprise! Where are you calling from?"

"I'm at the margii's house here in Ottawa. They said they haven't seen you for a while, so how are you doing?"

"I'm just fine, thank you, but this is incredible! The last time I saw you, we were having our kiirtan and meditation get-together at my place. It's been about thirty years since we've spoken."

"Yes, it's been a long time," he said. "So I was wondering if you'd like to come here for our kiirtan and meditation tomorrow afternoon?"

"Actually, I will be going to a spiritual centre near here tomorrow morning where I will be playing my drum during their service."

"Oh? Can I came with you?" he asked.

"Sure, dadaji! I think you'd enjoy the sermon and music, and it would be wonderful to see you again."

When I arrived at the centre the next morning, I mentioned to Rev. Nicole that an acarya would be coming to the service. She was delighted and said she would be happy to meet him.

"You can't miss him when he arrives," I said. "He'll be wearing his orange robe and turban."

I was using a cane temporarily because I had recently pulled a muscle in my left leg. So there I was hobbling along to the door as Rev. Nicole greeted him with outstretched arms. Dada paused for a moment as if not sure if it was me as I approached, which was rather comical, because at first glance I must have appeared much older leaning on the cane. Of course, after thirty years, time would have naturally taken its toll on us both.

But then I noticed our spirit hadn't waned any, our energy seemed as dynamic as ever. We did our namaskar salutations, and I led him to a seat I had saved next to David. Soft music played in the background, and we settled down, leaving any chatter until after the service. I looked around and saw there happened to be a medium sitting next to the podium where their guest speakers usually sit. They quite often had mediums who actually took part in the service. *Hum … dada might find this rather interesting,* I mused.

The medium was introduced near the end of the service, and as she began slowly walking up and down the aisles, she would stop and point at random to one of the people holding their hand up, indicating they would like to have a message. They were asked to stand and give their name, then the medium would give a message that came directly from a spirit—usually a loved one who wanted to make a connection. It just so happened that I also received a message along with the others that morning, which I found to be very interesting indeed.

"Women admire your strength of spirit," she said. "Your circle is complete."

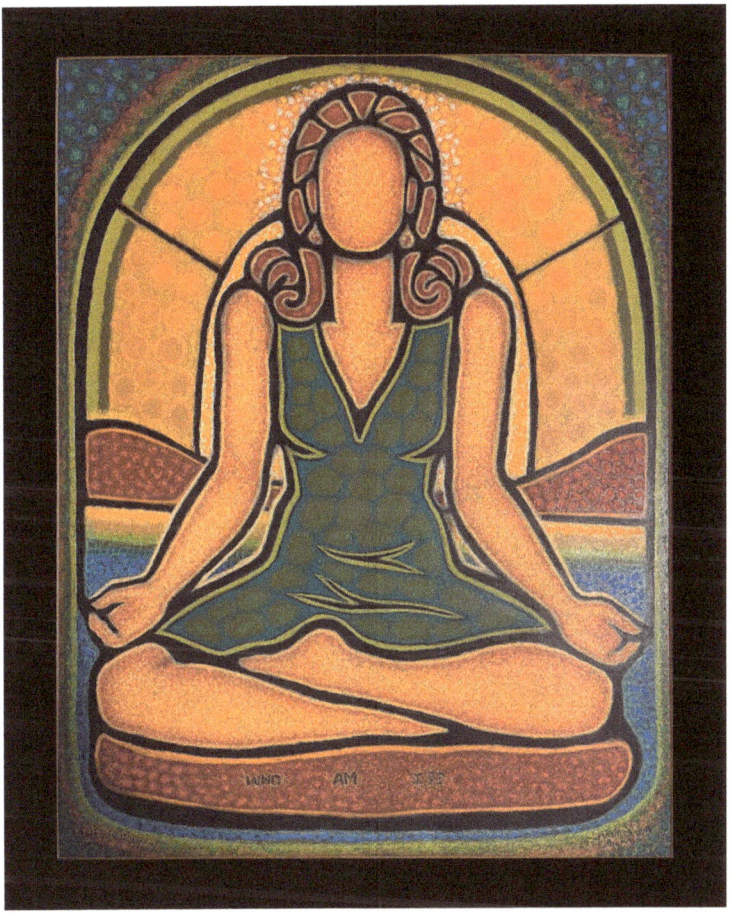

SELFREALIZATION

This meant that when I make my transition from this life (after having exhausted all my karmic reactions that I had come to live out), I will not have to take birth again in a physical form but will remain in the spiritual realm where I will continue to evolve in consciousness. She probably did half a dozen or more readings from among the forty or so of us who were in attendance that day.

We had decided that dada would stay with David and me for two days while he was in Ottawa. During that time, I recorded many devotional songs on my computer. He sang them for me, one right after another for two hours straight! I was amazed and appreciated him leaving this beautiful music with me. To this day, I often listen to the recordings while doing my spiritual practices first thing in the morning. It is such a wonderful way to start my day.

Just after dada left Ottawa, I talked to Rev. Nicole about our ancient spiritual dance called Akhanda Kiirtan. I explained how we move in a circle while singing our mantra, and she was quite intrigued. She wanted to find out more and even offered to make space in their program for it if we wanted to hold an event there some time. I mentioned this to dada in one of our short emails back and forth, and he said he'd make himself available if needed, but it would have to be in a couple of months' time because he was in Europe.

In the meantime, I asked a musician, Raul, who attended their services regularly if he'd be kind enough to play his guitar for the Akhanda Kiirtan. He said he'd be happy to, so he came to my place with his guitar. I gave him a tune I had made up, he wrote down the cords and we practised it a few times.

The following Sunday, he showed me the song sheet he had made with the cords and notes beautifully done. With that, I figured we were ready for the event. Rev. Nicole told me I had to say a few words before starting the dance to explain what it was about. This threw me for a loop because I had played only with margiis during akhanda kiirtans where everyone simply got up and began moving in the circle once the dance started. It made sense that someone should introduce the dance before it started, which would have to be me, of course.

It took a while, but I came up with a presentation that I hoped would explain it properly. When the time came to give that presentation, I was in my Anna Maria personality waiting for my turn to speak and knowing full well that I was not capable of doing this. *I could kick myself for putting myself in this position!* I thought. Just then, I heard Rev. Nicole say my name.

"Well, there's no backing down now," I muttered to myself.

Stepping up to the podium, my throat felt dry and my hands trembled slightly as I opened my folder.

"Good morning, everyone," I heard myself say as I glanced out over the audience.

I had this warm wave of peace pass through my entire being, and my mind suddenly became laser sharp, focusing 100% on every word of my presentation. I felt totally in control as if I had done this many times before. I couldn't believe what was happening as I stood there at the podium. It truly was an extraordinary experience. So much so that it changed my self-image from that day onward; I actually had confidence in myself that I had never known before.

So based on the positive response I received from the OSPC congregation, I decided to go to another multifaith centre to introduce this ancient spiritual dance. The next one, called Unity, was close to downtown. When I showed their reverend Roxanne the video of our Akhanda Kiirtan, she agreed to allow us to hold our dance at their centre. I then asked Spencer, the musician who was playing there at the time, if he'd be interested in participating. He was quite busy but still agreed to participate, knowing it would be as a service with no money involved.

When he came to my place with his guitar, I sang the tune I had in mind but noticed he hadn't written down any of the cords or notes. However, when it came time to play for the dance and everything went smoothly, I realized there was no reason for concern.

Our neighbours from India who lived directly across the hall from us had participated in the dance and said how much they enjoyed taking part.

"I have the video of today's Akhanda Kiirtan and thought you might like to see it," said David.

"Sure, thanks for bringing it over," Shibu responded.

When David opened the computer, my image appeared on the screen. I was opening my folder at the podium, about to give my presentation. What happened next was amazing. I was absolutely speechless as I stared at the screen. In those first few moments of that video, I had an instantaneous realization of what actually happened when I began to speak. For the first time, I saw myself in a personality other than Anna Maria (the one that everyone is familiar with). I realized it was actually my spiritual personality, Eta Purna, who had suddenly stepped in to give that presentation. Awestruck, I watched as she took over and immediately understood exactly what had transpired at that precise moment. I felt as if I was having some kind of out-of-body experience. Seeing for myself what transpired left me spellbound.

I don't know why I did not recognize this at the time it was happening to me. I thought I was the only one aware of the difference in my personalities as we watched that video, but David noticed it, too, as he pointed out later. Anyway, just before we left their apartment, I said, "I would like to put this Akhanda Kiirtan on YouTube, but I haven't a clue as to how to go about doing that."

"Oh, I can do that for you if you'd like," said Shibu.

"Are you kidding? Really?"

"No problem, I often do this sort of thing at work."

I was really surprised by his offer, and quite happy to leave the video there with him over the weekend. Around that time, I had been inspired by margiis from other parts of the world who had been posting their own videos and demonstrating other things, like a dance called kaoshiiki that was also given by our guru. This started me thinking about posting my own video as well. Shibu said he had taken a few clips from both videos and joined them together, but he needed a name or title to post it. I quickly came up with *Introducing Akhanda Kiirtan to Ottawa Spiritual Centres*.

In the meantime, I had let dada Sarvabodhananda know about our next Akhanda Kiirtan event in Ottawa, so he was able to come and play for us. I was elated because he had many beautiful kiirtan tunes he had picked up over time from wherever he was posted as an acarya in different countries. We only had a chance to hold a couple more of our Akhanda Kiirtan events before everything suddenly came to an abrupt halt with the onset of COVID-19.

We had to cancel our bookings at the spiritual centres, and dada and I ended up connecting mainly through short emails or an occasional phone call. Since that time, my contact with other spiritual aspirants has been via Zoom. It's been over two years since COVID-19 hit and, needless to say, this pandemic has changed everything in so many ways for everyone. It is unprecedented, and we have no way of knowing when or if it will ever disappear. So we're kind of left hanging when it comes to when we will be able get together again.

In the meantime, I continue with my spiritual practices, and I know this will never change. As always, I strive to maintain a balance on all levels—physical, mental and spiritual. David and I have been vaccinated for the coronavirus, and even though we've had our shots and were taking the necessary precautions, we still ended up with catching the omicron variant in 2022. He had it first and I caught a mild version two weeks later. We recently decided to get another booster shot.

There is still much to look forward to despite the many challenges coronavirus has placed before us, and we will get through this. I see light at the end of the tunnel.

Epilogue

David and I have every intention of making that trip back to Cape Breton to see Liz, Lynn and Andy. We will fly rather than take an RV this time, as I don't think there are many seniors in their eighties (David is eighty-two and I turned eighty in December) who relish the idea of driving long distances as we get up there in years.

Robert decided to drive to Cape Breton with his wife and two little girls for the first time a few years ago. Their plan was to spend their vacation there so that Robert would finally get to meet his brother, Andy, and his sister, Liz. When he finally made the trip, his girls were six and ten, and it was quite special for them to meet Andy, Liz and Lynn. I really appreciated Robert keeping in touch with me while he was there.

They gathered together in a designated spot and spent time getting to know a bit about each other. Before parting ways, Robert said they made plans to meet up again whenever possible in the future. I never understood why Stephen never showed interest in meeting his siblings. I thought he might be curious, but it just never happened. I was elated that Robert made the effort.

So here we are in 2022. I started to write this book in January 2020, two months before the coronavirus arrived on the scene. As I read over what I have written thus far, I see I have covered most of the traumas that have impacted my life as well as many of the pivotal moments since my journey began back in December of 1942. However, there are a couple of incidents that I just could not bring myself to talk about. Even with the passing of time (over fifty years), I am still not able to go there in my mind.

As we enter this last phase of our lives, David and I are closer than we have ever been. Since we both happen to be homebodies, we are content just being together after a busy day. He has often remarked how peaceful it is to come in from work and find me meditating with soft music in the background. He sits and absorbs the calm vibration while having his usual little snack.

Come to think of it, we haven't been apart since I moved to Ottawa to be with him in 2006. He recently spent five days in the hospital when he suddenly came down with shingles, which has left him with nerve pain in his back, but he is slowly on the mend. It's remarkable that he is still working at the age of eighty-two, but he will have to step back at some point, regardless of how much he enjoys connecting with many people there at work. I'm pretty sure he'll appreciate having some time for himself when he finally does let go of the reins. He has often remarked that he'd like to have more time to read, for example. He has been an avid reader all his life and he has such an inquisitive mind that always keeps him busy, so he will be quite satisfied when he takes that next inevitable step.

Our little Munchkin cat is still with us and is more affectionate than ever in his old age. I was talking to our vet the other day, and she said, "When I look at his chart, I can hardly believe he'll be nineteen years old in a month's time. His health problems are so few in comparison to most of the others at our cat hospital." I read that the lifespan of the Munchkin breed is normally fifteen years, so every year beyond is a bonus. He has been my constant companion over the years, and I love him dearly.

However, there is something he doesn't seem to understand: that we humans need our sleep at night! He has this habit of jumping up onto the bed and slowly creeping over to see if I'm awake. He then gives a little meow while staring down into my face, and if I don't respond, he ever so gently nips at my arm, as if to say, "Put your arm around me! I want to snuggle." If I don't respond (which happens sometimes), he bunts me with his head and continues to nip at my arm until I can't help but react—he's just so adorable.

Another thing Munchkin does is visit our neighbour's cat named Bob, who is also black and white but is much bigger, with a rather lanky look about him as he glides by. He's the nervous type, so Munchkin often has to coax him to come in. With both of them being indoor cats, our neighbour and I leave our doors open a few inches so they can feel free to visit each other during the day.

"Munchkin sure talks a lot doesn't he!" the neighbour remarked one time.

Sometimes when he wants Bob to follow him back to our apartment, he calls him with a loud, slightly high-pitched meow (as if calling his name). Bob peeks out to make sure no one else is in the hall before he comes trailing behind. Then Munchkin coaches him along with a deeper tone when he reaches our door, as if saying, "Come on, Bob, it's okay." Bob never stays very long, unlike Munchkin who spends quite a bit of time over at Bob's.

Once in a while, I catch the two of them having what I call a boxing match. All of a sudden, they start hitting each other through the small space where the door is left open. I will hear a sort of rattle at the door and turn to see Bob's long paw reaching in to hit Munchkin, whose short little paws are rapidly striking back. This lasts only about six seconds or so, then Munchkin suddenly stops. With his lion-like stride, he walks away with an air of superiority as if to say, "There! I won THAT round!" It's so comical and cute.

Bob quickly disappears but always comes back later looking for Munchkin, who is usually curled up in a ball on the recliner by then. It is such a pleasure to have these little guys around; they are like members of the family and we treat them as such.

It doesn't concern me at all that time is running out and I won't be here much longer in this physical form. This is probably because of my understanding that the mind doesn't actually stop once it leaves the body. We continue on in consciousness after making our transition where we will have the opportunity to move forward in our evolution of consciousness.

After spending these last three years outlining the twists and turns of my life's journey, I have concluded that the time was well spent. It has helped me gain insight and a deeper understanding of who I truly am. That I am NOT the worthless individual I had always thought myself to be because of wrong messages my mind held onto from childhood. After years of soul-searching, I have discovered that in times of despair, the only escape is to go within. It's where I finally found the peace of mind I had been searching for and the understanding I am an eternal soul (as we all are) and will one day merge back into the cosmic consciousness (God) from which we came. This belief has helped me through the ups and downs of life and continues to do so as I move closer to my goal with each passing day.

There is something I'd like to leave with you as I say goodbye. I put these few words together just a few days ago while in a rather contemplative mood:

Loving words are POWERFUL. They can heal the heart and mind.

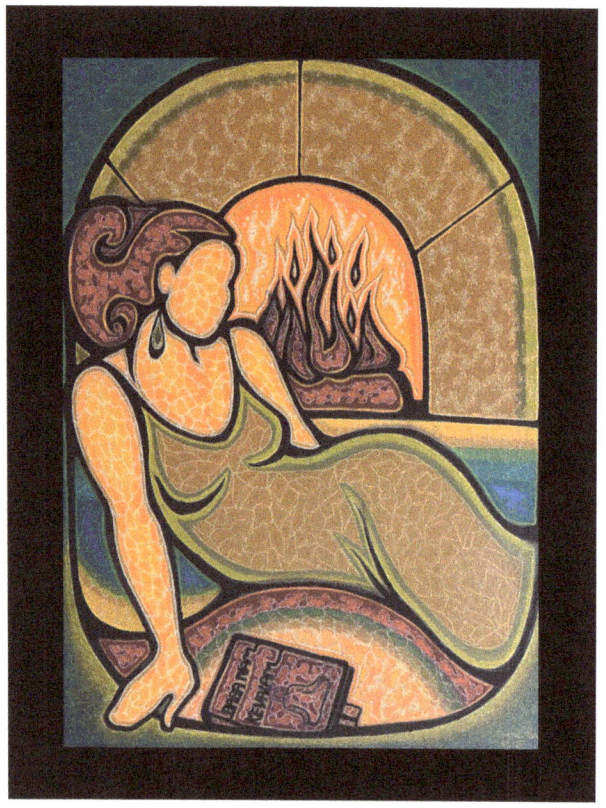

FIRESIDE EVENING

I also have this little poem I wrote back in the late 1970s that I would like to share with you as well.

Be Always with Me

I want to feel you always with me
In everything I do
Your presence is so precious
As a gift of love I cherish and hold dear
When we're alone, there is no time
As you ease my mind with thoughts of you
Letting me know you're always here
Not only in this way
But through others you put me with throughout the day
in this endless "liila," your cosmic play.

by devotee Amrta (Anna Maria Scott)

In closing, I sincerely wish everyone finds the lasting peace and happiness that is deep within your soul—that spark of divinity which is exactly the same in each and every one of us.

Namaskar (salutation meaning "I respect the divinity within you").

Acknowledgment

A special thank you to the entire Tellwell team; especially to those who gave extra support during the publishing process.

www.ingramcontent.com/pod-product-compliance
Lightning Source LLC
LaVergne TN
LVHW051225070526
838200LV00057B/4601